Laboratory Monitoring of Gastrointestinal and Hepatobiliary Disease

Editor

STANLEY J. NAIDES

GASTROENTEROLOGY CLINICS OF NORTH AMERICA

www.gastro.theclinics.com

Consulting Editor
ALAN L. BUCHMAN

June 2019 • Volume 48 • Number 2

ELSEVIER

1600 John F. Kennedy Boulevard • Suite 1800 • Philadelphia, Pennsylvania, 19103-2899
http://www.theclinics.com

GASTROENTEROLOGY CLINICS OF NORTH AMERICA Volume 48, Number 2
June 2019 ISSN 0889-8553, ISBN-13: 978-0-323-67870-4

Editor: Kerry Holland
Developmental Editor: Laura Kavanaugh

Gastroenterology Clinics of North America (ISSN 0889-8553) is published quarterly by Elsevier Inc., 360 Park Avenue South, New York, NY 10010-1710. Months of issue are March, June, September, and December. Business and Editorial Offices: 1600 John F. Kennedy Blvd., Suite 1800, Philadelphia, PA 19103-2899. Customer Service Office: 6277 Sea Harbor Drive, Orlando, FL 32887-4800. Periodicals postage paid at New York, NY and additional mailing offices. Subscription prices are $361.00 per year (US individuals), $100.00 per year (US students), $692.00 per year (US institutions), $387.00 per year (Canadian individuals), $220.00 per year (Canadian students), $849.00 per year (Canadian institutions), $463.00 per year (international individuals), $220.00 per year (international students), and $849.00 per year (international institutions). Foreign air speed delivery is included in all *Clinics* subscription prices. All prices are subject to change without notice. **POSTMASTER:** Send address changes to *Gastroenterology Clinics of North America*, Elsevier Health Sciences Division, Subscription Customer Service, 3251 Riverport Lane, Maryland Heights, MO 63043. **Telephone: 1-800-654-2452 (U.S. and Canada); 314-447-8871 (outside U.S. and Canada). Fax: 314-447-8029. E-mail: journalscustomerservice-usa@elsevier.com (for print support); journalsonlinesupport-usa@elsevier.com (for online support).**

Reprints. For copies of 100 or more, of articles in this publication, please contact the Commercial Reprints Department, Elsevier Inc., 360 Part Avenue South, New York, New York 10010-1710. Tel. 212-633-3874, Fax: 212-633-3820, E-mail: reprints@elsevier.com.

Gastroenterology Clinics of North America is also published in Italian by Il Pensiero Scientifico Editore, Rome, Italy; and in Portuguese by Interlivros Edicoes Ltda., Rua Commandante Coelho 1085, 21250 Cordovil, Rio de Janeiro, Brazil.

Gastroenterology Clinics of North America is covered in *MEDLINE/PubMed (Index Medicus), Excerpta Medica, Current Contents/Clinical Medicine, Science Citation Index, ISI/BIOMED,* and *BIOSIS.*

Contributors

CONSULTING EDITOR

ALAN L. BUCHMAN, MD, MSPH, FACP, FACN, FACG, AGAF
Medical Director, Health Care Services Corporation, Professor of Clinical Surgery and Medical Director, Intestinal Rehabilitation and Transplant Center, The University of Illinois at Chicago, Chicago, Illinois, USA

EDITOR

STANLEY J. NAIDES, MD
Formerly, Medical Director, Immunology R&D, Quest Diagnostics Nichols Institute, San Juan Capistrano, Currently, President, Stanley J. Naides, MD, PC, Dana Point, California

AUTHORS

NEZAM H. AFDHAL, MD
Professor, Department of Medicine, Liver Center, Beth Israel Deaconess Medical Center, Harvard Medical School, Boston, Massachusetts, USA

KENNETH I. BERNS, MD, PhD
Department of Molecular Genetics and Microbiology, Powell Gene Therapy Center, Distinguished Professor Emeritus, University of Florida College of Medicine, Gainesville, Florida, USA

DAVID E. ELLIOTT, MD, PhD
Professor, Department of Internal Medicine, Division of Gastroenterology and Hepatology, University of Iowa, Carver College of Medicine, Staff Physician, Iowa City VA Health Care System, Iowa City, Iowa, USA

SARAH GLOVER, DO
Associate Professor, University of Florida Health, Gainesville, Florida, USA

RUBEN BONILLA GUERRERO, MD
Admera Health, South Plainfield, New Jersey, USA

COLIN HILL, MSc, PhD, DSc
School of Microbiology, APC Microbiome Ireland, University College Cork, Cork, Ireland

M. NEDIM INCE, MD
Assistant Professor, Department of Internal Medicine, Division of Gastroenterology and Hepatology, University of Iowa, Carver College of Medicine, Staff Physician, Iowa City VA Health Care System, Iowa City, Iowa, USA

AREZOU KHOSROSHAHI, MD
Associate Professor, Department of Medicine, Emory University, Atlanta, Georgia, USA

KAREN M. KLOKE, MS
Mayo Clinic, Rochester, Minnesota, USA

MICHELLE LAI, MD, MPH
Assistant Professor, Department of Medicine, Liver Center, Beth Israel Deaconess Medical Center, Harvard Medical School, Boston, Massachusetts, USA

AONGHUS LAVELLE, MB, PhD
Department of Medicine, APC Microbiome Ireland, University College Cork, Cork, Ireland

AARON LERNER, MD, MHA
B. Rappaport School of Medicine, Technion-Israel Institute of Technology, Haifa, Israel; AESKU.KIPP Institute, Wendelsheim, Germany

TORSTEN MATTHIAS, PhD
AESKU.KIPP Institute, Wendelsheim, Germany

KUNATUM PRASIDTHRATHSINT, MD
Division of Infectious Diseases, Department of Internal Medicine, Division of Clinical Microbiology, Department of Pathology, Department of Microbiology and Immunology, University of Iowa Carver College of Medicine, University of Iowa Hospitals and Clinics, Iowa City, Iowa, USA

AJAY RAMESH, PhD
AESKU.KIPP Institute, Wendelsheim, Germany

DENISE SALAZAR, PhD
Quest Diagnostics, San Juan Capistrano, California, USA

DAVID SCHWIMMER, MD
Gastroenterology Fellow, University of Florida Health, Gainesville, Florida, USA

ARUN SRIVASTAVA, PhD
Division of Cellular and Molecular Therapy, Departments of Pediatrics, and Molecular Genetics and Microbiology, Powell Gene Therapy Center, Cancer and Genetics Research Complex, George H. Kitzman Professor of Genetics, University of Florida College of Medicine, Gainesville, Florida, USA

JACK T. STAPLETON, MD
Professor, Division of Infectious Diseases, Department of Internal Medicine, Department of Microbiology and Immunology, University of Iowa Carver College of Medicine, University of Iowa Hospitals and Clinics, Medicine and Research Services, Iowa City VA Health Care Center, Iowa City, Iowa

BIJAL VASHI, MD
Rheumatology Fellow, Department of Medicine, Emory University, Atlanta, Georgia, USA

Contents

Inborn errors of metabolism (IEMs) are usually recognized by character-istic neurologic and metabolic manifestations and sometimes by dysmorphism. However, IEMs can present with a wide variety of gastro-intestinal manifestations, whether as the primary or a minor clinical symptom. Regardless, gastrointestinal and hepatic manifestations of IEMs are important clinical features that can help identify an underlying defect; these disorders should be taken into consideration as part of a patient's clinical assessment. It is prudent to include metabolic disorders in the differential diagnosis because in some cases, gastrointestinal symptoms may be the only presenting feature in a patient with an under-lying IEM.

This article presents the most common gastrointestinal, hepatic, and pancreatic manifestations of the primary immunodeficiency diseases, including the appropriate laboratory testing, endoscopic evaluation, and recommendations for further management.

The gut microbiome is fundamental to human health and development. Altered microbiomes have been associated with many diseases. However, variation between individuals, environmental effects, and a lack of stan-dardization across studies makes differentiation between health and dis-ease challenging. Large-scale population cohorts in different countries will be required to match disease subjects with healthy controls, whereas standardized, reproducible pipelines for analysis are required to compare findings between studies. Despite this, several conditions have already demonstrated great promise for developing microbiome-based bio-markers as well as providing a gateway into integrated personalized medicine.

Inflammatory bowel disease (IBD) comprises a group of chronic, intestinal inflammatory disorders, including ulcerative colitis and Crohn's disease. IBD is characterized by periods of relapse and remission. Long-term progressive intestinal inflammation can result in severe and devastating complications, such as intestinal strictures and/or fistulae. Immune suppressive medications with potent side effects are often used to control inflammation and limit disease activity. Laboratory tests guide various decisions in clinical management of IBD. We discuss tests used to diagnose IBD, assess for relapse or remission, monitor the effectiveness of therapeutic regimen, screen for the maintenance of health, and diagnose or prevent complications.

Many microbes, toxins, autoimmune diseases, and neoplastic diseases may cause liver inflammation; however, 5 viruses whose main pathogenesis is liver disease are referred to as hepatitis A, B, C, D, and E viruses. These viruses cause a significant burden of global illness. With the exception of hepatitis A virus, all may cause chronic infection potentially leading to cirrhosis and hepatocellular carcinoma. Excellent serologic and nucleic acid detection methods are available for determining the precise cause and, in some cases, the duration of infection. Diagnostics are critical for identifying individuals needing treatment and for monitoring the treatment success.

All chronic liver disease can lead to liver fibrosis. Assessment of the severity of liver fibrosis is central to making treatment and management decisions. Liver biopsy, the gold standard for liver fibrosis assessment, is invasive and carries risks of complications and sampling errors. The use of noninvasive elastography-based radiologic methods of liver fibrosis determination is limited to centers that have the capabilities. Laboratory liver fibrosis determinations, both general clinical scoring systems and combination biomarker panels, are accessible to a wider population of clinicians for identifying patients at low risk of advanced fibrosis who do not need liver biopsies.

IgG4-related disease is an immune-mediated fibroinflammatory condition with a diverse spectrum of organ involvement, commonly in the pancreas and bile ducts among other organs such as salivary and lacrimal glands. Classic histopathologic findings are the gold standard for confirmation of diagnosis, although diagnosis remains challenging, as biomarkers to date are neither sufficient nor necessary. Glucocorticoids are the most effective initial treatment, generally having a dramatic response, although limited clinical evidence exists regarding effective maintenance therapy. This review summarizes key GI manifestations of this condition for the practicing gastroenterologist and addresses the pathology, disease mechanism, and current therapeutic recommendations.

Most patients affected by celiac disease (CD) are asymptomatic or hyposymptomatic and undiagnosed, and are at risk of preventable complications. Therefore, early diagnosis is highly recommended. Multiple diagnostic antibodies are available; the most frequently used is IgA to tissue transglutaminase (IgA-tTg). It may yield false results and, alone, does not address IgA deficiency. Recently, a new generation of anti-neo-epitope tTg check (IgG + IgA) has become available. It is highly sensitive and specific, covers IgA-deficient patients with CD, reflects intestinal damage, and has predictive potential in the diagnosis of CD.

Recombinant vectors based on a nonpathogenic parvovirus, the adeno-associated virus (AAV), have taken center stage in the past decade. The safety of AAV vectors in clinical trials and clinical efficacy in several human diseases are now well documented. Despite these achievements, it is increasingly clear that the full potential of AAV vectors composed of the naturally occurring capsids is unlikely to be realized. This article describes advances that have been made and challenges that remain in the optimal use of AAV vectors in human gene therapy applications.

GASTROENTEROLOGY
CLINICS OF NORTH AMERICA

SERIES OF RELATED INTEREST

Gastrointestinal Endoscopy Clinics of North America
(Available at: https://www.giendo.theclinics.com)
Clinics in Liver Disease
(Available at: https://www.liver.theclinics.com)

THE CLINICS ARE AVAILABLE ONLINE!
Access your subscription at:
www.theclinics.com

Foreword

The Laboratory in Gastroenterology: Use and Abuse

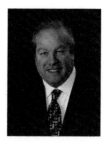

Alan L. Buchman, MD, MSPH, FACP, FACN, FACG, AGAF
Consulting Editor

It's not just the gastrointestinal/endoscopy lab that's important in the diagnosis and treatment as well as determining disease course in gastroenterology, it's the chemistry and physiology laboratory. This laboratory must be effectively and appropriately utilized for the correct indications. As testing has become increasingly sophisticated and individualized, so must our thinking evolve. The emphasis though remains on utilizing the laboratory to make a difference in clinical management; in today's times it's not sufficient just to know. We all know the laboratory is useful in diagnostics, but it has evolved to create therapies as well. The laboratory will help us to understand better the relationship between genetics and our environment; food and the microbiome, which may regulate nutritional status, yet in turn be itself regulated by diet, disease, and/or genetics, and in a further permutation, the microbiome may modulate genetics and cause or modulate disease activity. The modern laboratory is emerging as the backbone behind "personalized" medicine and risk management.

In this issue of *Gastroenterology Clinics of North America*, Dr Stanley Naides has assembled an outstanding and diverse group of individuals who have developed or are experts in the use of a variety of laboratory testing procedures for various diseases and conditions that the gastroenterologist will encounter in either children or adults. Dr

Gastroenterol Clin N Am 48 (2019) ix–x
https://doi.org/10.1016/j.gtc.2019.04.001
0889-8553/19/© 2019 Published by Elsevier Inc.

Naides himself has made a career in the development and validation of scaled up laboratory testing.

Alan L. Buchman, MD, MSPH, FACP, FACN, FACG, AGAF
Intestinal Rehabilitation and Transplant Center
Department of Surgery
College of Medicine
The University of Illinois at Chicago 8
40 South Wood Street
Suite 402 Clinical Sciences Building
MC 958
Chicago, IL 60612, USA

Health Care Services Corporation
300 East Randolph Street
Chicago, IL 60601, USA

E-mail address:
buchman@uic.edu

Preface

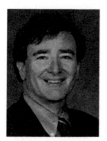

Stanley J. Naides, MD
Editor

The clinical laboratory plays a critical, central role in the diagnosis, prognosis, and management of patients with gastrointestinal and liver diseases. Progress in understanding disease pathogenesis, improved test methodologies, and identification of clinically relevant biomarkers has made the laboratory's contributions to clinical practice all the more integral to quality patient care. The laboratory's role in promoting personalized medicine is foundational.

Despite the importance of the laboratory to clinical practice, the trend in medical education has been away from providing laboratory hands-on experience.[1,2] Such experience allows learners to understand nuances in testing methods, quality control and assurance, and test result interpretation, but these lessons require student laboratory space, blocks for teaching time, and integration into the curriculum.[2-4] Investment in medical student teaching in laboratory medicine yields long-term benefit in terms of wise test ordering and cost-effective care.[5,6] Curriculum developers are challenged by the explosion in medical knowledge and are often forced to choose among competing educational needs.[7]

At the medical residency level, the days of the ward satellite laboratory, where interns personally reviewed urine sediment, peripheral blood smears, Gram stains, and acid-fast stains, are long since gone.[8,9] So too are the days when the housestaff had to venture to the clinical laboratory to discuss histology and laboratory results with laboratory personnel and the hospital pathologist if they wanted test results in a timely fashion. These exertions have been obviated as a consequence of the Clinical Laboratory Improvement Act, centralization, outsourcing of testing, and computerized resulting to the bedside.[10-12]

Fellowship training has also been affected by a trend away from laboratory training. There are fewer divisional laboratories performing basic laboratory research as a consequence of tighter federal funding for basic science research. Investigators have turned to industry funding that supports clinical outcomes and drug therapy trials. Despite the changes in the training environment, fellows learn well the application of laboratory results to the patients they see, but the need to better bridge the divide between the laboratory and the clinic remains.

Gastroenterol Clin N Am 48 (2019) xi–xiii
https://doi.org/10.1016/j.gtc.2019.03.001
0889-8553/19/© 2019 Published by Elsevier Inc.

gastro.theclinics.com

This issue is a contribution to bringing the laboratory to the clinic. Drs Bonilla-Guererro, Kloke, and Salazar discuss the gastrointestinal and hepatic presentations of inborn errors of metabolism, providing broader differential diagnostic considerations, even when there is minimal or no metabolic decompensation. Drs Schwimmer and Glover review the infectious and autoimmune complications of primary immunodeficiencies that physicians are likely to encounter. Drs Lai and Afdahl describe the various laboratory biomarkers and algorithms as well as newer ultrasound techniques used to stage liver fibrosis. Drs Ince and Elliott review the role of the laboratory in the diagnosis and management of inflammatory bowel disease. The A, B, Cs (and D and E) of viral hepatitis are reviewed by Drs Prasidthrathsint and Stapleton. Drs Vashi and Khosroshahi describe the newly recognized immunoglobulin IgG4-related disease, highlighting the gastrointestinal manifestations. The exciting field of bowel microbiome studies is reviewed by Drs Lavelle and Hill. Drs Lerner, Ajay, and Torsten update new approaches to the laboratory diagnosis of an old disease, celiac disease. Finally, gene therapy to treat liver dysfunction is currently being brought to the clinic, and Drs Berns and Srivastava describe the role of adenovirus-associated virus vector delivery in realizing the promise of gene therapy.

We hope that the reader will find this issue informative and that it will promote understanding of how the laboratory can contribute to patient care. Perhaps it will prompt the reader to reach across the divide: the clinician to pick up the telephone to call the laboratorian or visit the local laboratory to sit down with the clinical pathologist to discuss a case, and conversely, for the laboratorian to reach out to clinical colleagues to learn about the provider's experience and the patient's journey.

Stanley J. Naides, MD
33072 Sunharbor Dana Point, CA 92629, USA

E-mail address:
stanley.naides@gmail.com

REFERENCES

1. Gottfried EL, Kamoun M, Burke MD. Laboratory medicine education in United States medical schools. Am J Clin Pathol 1993;100:594–8.

2. Smith BR, Kamoun M, Hickner J. Laboratory medicine education at US medical schools: a 2014 status report. Acad Med 2016;91:107–12.

3. Delfiner MS, Martinez LR, Pavia CS. A gram stain hands-on workshop enhances first year medical students' technique competency in comprehension and memorization. PLoS One 2016;11:e0163658.

4. Carbo AR, Blanco PG, Graeme-Cooke F, et al. Revitalizing pathology laboratories in a gastrointestinal pathophysiology course using multimedia and team-based learning techniques. Pathol Res Pract 2012;208:300–5.

5. Yamanaka M. [A need for undergraduate education for laboratory medicine in medical schools]. Rinsho Byori 1996;44:709–14 [in Japanese].

6. Bennett BD, Gardner WA Jr. Teaching laboratory medicine. The clinical laboratory experience. Arch Pathol Lab Med 1986;110:978–9.

7. Smith BR, Aguero-Rosenfeld M, Anastasi J, et al, Academy of Clinical Laboratory Physicians and Scientists. Educating medical students in laboratory medicine: a proposed curriculum. Am J Clin Pathol 2010;133:533–42.

8. Fine MJ, Orloff JJ, Rihs JD, et al. Evaluation of housestaff physicians' preparation and interpretation of sputum gram stains for community-acquired pneumonia. J Gen Intern Med 1991;6:189–98.

9. Peredy TR, Powers RD. Bedside diagnostic testing of body fluids. Am J Emerg Med 1997;15:400–7.

10. Lee-Lewandrowski E, Lewandrowski K. Regulatory compliance for point-of-care testing. A perspective from the United States (circa 2000). Clin Lab Med 2001; 21:241–53, vii.

11. Fischer S, Stewart TE, Mehta S, et al. Handheld computing in medicine. J Am Med Inform Assoc 2003;10:139–49.

12. Strom CS. Changing trends in laboratory testing in the United States. Clin Lab Med 2012;32:651–64.

Inborn Errors of Metabolism and the Gastrointestinal Tract

Ruben Bonilla Guerrero, MD[a],*, Karen M. Kloke, MS[b],
Denise Salazar, PhD[c]

KEYWORDS

- Gastrointestinal • Hepatic • Manifestations • Inborn • Error • Metabolism • Disorder

KEY POINTS

- Inborn errors of metabolism should be included in the differential diagnosis when facing a patient with gastrointestinal manifestations, even with minimal or no metabolic decompensation.
- The type of gastrointestinal manifestation can narrow down the potential underlying inborn errors of metabolism.
- There are multiple mechanisms by which gastrointestinal pathophysiology can occur in inherited metabolic defects.

INTRODUCTION

Inborn errors of metabolism (IEMs) are a group of inherited disorders in which molecular abnormalities occur in genes related to metabolic pathways, most often leading to enzymatic deficiencies that disrupt the body's normal metabolic processes. When a metabolic step is blocked, the substrates of the affected enzyme build up and, in some cases, enter alternate metabolic pathways that are not utilized or are underutilized in normal circumstances; some of these intermediate metabolites are toxic at high levels, either directly or indirectly, and can affect multiple organ systems. This article focuses on IEMs that are known to have gastrointestinal (GI) manifestations, because these disorders should be considered in a patient's differential diagnosis.

Persistent GI complaints represent diagnostic challenges for physicians because they can be found in many common disorders, such as celiac disease or irritable

Disclosure Statement: The authors do not have any relationship with a commercial company that has a direct financial interest in subject matter or materials discussed in article or with a company making a competing product.
[a] Admera Health, 126 Corporate Boulevard, South Plainfield, NJ 07080, USA; [b] Mayo Clinic, 200 First Street Southwest, Rochester, MN 55905, USA; [c] Quest Diagnostics, 33608 Ortega Highway, San Juan Capistrano, CA 92690, USA
* Corresponding author.
E-mail address: ruben.b.guerrero@admerahealth.com

bowel syndrome. Even when more common causes have been ruled out, IEMs are not typically considered when GI manifestations are the primary presenting symptom. A range of GI findings can be observed in IEMs, including recurrent abdominal pain, chronic vomiting, acute pancreatitis, chronic diarrhea, constipation, and malabsorption. Because these presenting features are relatively nonspecific, a patient may be misdiagnosed or remain undiagnosed for many years, during which quality of life may be significantly impacted.

IEMs that present with chronic diarrhea and failure to thrive can be divided into disorders effecting the intestinal mucosa itself and systemic disorders. Disorders of the intestinal mucosa that yield almost exclusively intestinal symptoms include hereditary folate malabsorption, transcobalamin II deficiency, glucose/galactose malabsorption, sucrase-isomaltase deficiency, congenital chloride diarrhea, and Pearson syndrome, among others (**Table 1**).

ABDOMINAL PAIN

Abdominal pain is a hallmark symptom for several IEMs, although an underlying metabolic disease may not be considered in the differential diagnosis until after several recurrences, thereby delaying diagnosis. Typical abdominal pain associated with IEMs is diffuse and often intense, and its severity may lead to surgical exploration for suspected gall bladder crisis or appendicitis. A few disorders that present with diffuse abdominal pain are discussed, with a more complete listing given in **Table 2**.

Acute Porphyrias

The acute hepatic porphyrias are inborn errors of heme metabolism which, unlike most enzyme defects, follow an autosomal dominant inheritance pattern. Deficiencies of enzymes in the heme biosynthetic pathway lead to the accumulation of heme precursors, some of which have neurotoxic properties. Because these are dominant disorders, clinical features often are not observed until aggravating factors, such as drugs, alcohol, illness, or steroid hormonal changes affect the body's requirement for heme. Acute intermittent porphyria (AIP), hereditary coproporphyria (HCP), and variegate porphyria (VP) all are acute porphyrias with similar clinical presentations. Of the 3, AIP is the most common, although only approximately 10% to 20% of individuals carrying a disease-causing variant ever develop clinical symptoms.[1]

One hallmark clinical presentation of the acute hepatic porphyrias is acute abdominal pain; it is present in up to 95% of cases and is usually accompanied by nausea, vomiting, abdominal distention and guarding, diarrhea, or constipation. These manifestations may lead to hyponatremia and, less frequently, to hypochloremia and hypomagnesemia. In addition to GI symptoms, patients may experience extremity pain, paresthesia, and mental disturbances, including changes in mental status, hallucinations, anxiety, depression, confusion, and seizures; the neurologic symptoms are most likely secondary to increased levels of the neurotoxic porphyrin precursors aminolevulinic acid (ALA) and porphobilinogen. Although cutaneous photosensitivity is not seen in AIP, approximately 20% of HCP patients and 80% of VP experience skin fragility and bullous lesions after exposure to sunlight. The intermittent nature of the clinical symptoms combined with the psychiatric presentations initially may lead to the suspicion of a psychosomatic disorder. In general, girls and women are more likely to experience clinical symptoms, with onset typically between the second and fourth decades of life, consistent with monthly hormonal changes; however, diagnosis is often delayed by a decade or more.[2]

Laboratory findings in the porphyrias include elevated urinary porphobilinogen and ALA as well as a pattern of elevated porphyrins specific to the affected enzymatic step. Urine specimens should be collected during a symptomatic episode whenever possible, because analyte levels may resolve to normal during quiescent periods. In most cases, a random urine sample is acceptable, although there can be significant diurnal variation in the excretion of porphyrins in girls and women.[3,4] Although plasma porphyrin levels can range from normal to mildly elevated in these cases, fecal porphyrins analysis aids in distinguishing between the 3 main acute porphyrias, because protoporphyrin, which is increased in cases of VP, is not detected in urine due to its limited solubility.[5]

Tyrosinemia Type I

Tyrosinemia type I is an autosomal recessive inherited defect in the distal portion of the tyrosine degradative pathway that prevents the hydrolysis of fumarylacetoacetate to fumarate and acetoacetate. The blocked enzymatic step in the breakdown of tyrosine leads to its buildup in tissues and organs. There are 3 types of tyrosinemia arising from defects in different enzymes in the shared pathway, but type I is the most severe. Clinical symptoms begin within the first few months of life with failure to thrive. Infants poorly tolerate high-protein foods, and their ingestion may lead to diarrhea and vomiting. Other clinical findings include hepatomegaly, splenomegaly, cirrhosis, liver failure, tubulopathy, nephromegaly, Fanconi syndrome, and seizures. Some affected patients have neurologic symptoms originating from an increase in succinylacetone formed from the accumulated fumarylacetoacetate; succinylacetone is a competitive inhibitor of ALA dehydratase, the first enzyme in the heme synthetic pathway, leading to an increase in ALA. These recurrent crises mimic those seen in the acute porphyrias with abdominal pain, peripheral neuropathy, changes in mental status, and potential respiratory failure.[6] Laboratory findings include elevated urinary succinylacetone seen in urine organic acid analysis, increased urinary ALA, and elevated plasma tyrosine and methionine.

Fabry Disease

Fabry disease is a lysosomal storage disorder resulting from a deficiency of α-galactosidase. It commonly presents with nonspecific GI symptoms, such as abdominal pain, distension, nausea, vomiting, constipation and diarrhea; these symptoms appear early in the disease progression, usually during childhood. Abdominal pain is one of the most commonly reported GI findings and has been described as a burning pain with superficial abdominal skin tenderness and discomfort. Symptoms may be exacerbated by stress or changes in diet and may worsen within minutes of eating, which may make the patient reluctant to eat. Diarrhea also is common, noted in approximately 20% of patients. Episodes may be related to food intake and can be frequent, with as many as 12 defecations per day. Conversely, constipation also is found, although less frequently and primarily in female patients. Other GI manifestations include early satiety, gastroparesis, gastritis or ulcer, hemorrhoids, pseudo-obstruction, bowel ischemia, diverticulitis, and pancreatitis.[7]

VOMITING

Organic acidurias, urea cycle disorders with hyperammonemia, and fatty acid oxidation defects are among the IEMs where vomiting is a characteristic feature. Chronic vomiting is seen during acidotic episodes of propionic aciduria, methylmalonic aciduria, and isovaleric aciduria; the isovaleryl–coenzyme A (CoA) that accumulates in isovaleric acidemia and the propionyl-CoA that accumulates in methylmalonic and

Table 1
Disorders with chronic diarrhea, poor feeding, failure to thrive

Additional GI Manifestations	Other Symptoms	Disorder and Subtype	Enzyme/Defect	Gene	Age of Onset	Laboratory Testing
Severe watery diarrhea Dehydration	Hypochloremia Hypokalemia Metabolic alkalosis	Congenital chloride diarrhea	Electrolyte disorder	SLC26A3	Congenital Neonatal	Electrolytes
	Reducing substances in feces	Glucose galactose malabsorption	SGLT1 deficiency	SGLT1	Neonatal	Urine glucose Glucose tolerance test Fructose tolerance test
	Bullous skin lesions Alopecia Nail dystrophy	Acrodermatitis enteropathica	Zinc deficiency	SLC39A4	Neonatal	Zinc levels Alkaline phosphatase
Vomiting Proteinuria Hepatomegaly	Fibrous of the liver Coagulation abnormalities Hypoglycemia	Congenital disorder of glycosylation (CDG) type 1b	Phosphomannose isomerase	MPI	Infancy	Plasma transferrin Enzyme testing
	Coagulation abnormalities Hypoglycemia	Congenital disorder of glycosylation (CDG) type 1h	α3-Glucosyl transferase	ALG8	Infancy	
Severe failure to thrive Anorexia Poor feeding	Frequent infections Lymphopenia Progressive neurologic symptoms	Adenosine deaminase deficiency	Adenosine deaminase	ADA	Neonatal to infancy	Gammaglobulin White blood cell count

Clinical features	Disease	Defect	Gene	Age of onset	Investigations
Severe failure to thrive, Anorexia, Poor feeding, With megaloblastic anemia					
Oral lesions, Neuropathy, Pancytopenia, Homocystinuria, Methylmalonic aciduria	Transcobalamin II deficiency	Defect of vitamin B12 transport	TCN2	Neonate	Urine organic acids, Plasma amino acids, Vitamin B12
Stomatitis, Neuropathy, Infections, Immune deficiency	Hereditary folate malabsorption	Impaired folate absorption and transport	SLC46A1	Infancy	Folate
Pancytopenia, Lactic acidosis, Pancreatic dysfunction	Pearson syndrome	Mitochondrial disorder	contiguous gene deletion/duplication syndrome involving several mtDNA genes	Neonate	Urine organic acids, Lactic acid, Plasma amino acids
Severe failure to thrive, Anorexia, Poor feeding, With predominant hepato-splenomegaly					
Irritable bowel syndrome, Hyper-IgD	Mevalonic aciduria	Mevalonate kinase	MVK	Infancy	Urine organic acids, IgD, Transaminases, Serum bile acids
Inflammatory bowel disease, Severe hypoglycemia	Glycogen storage disease type Ib	Glucose-6-phosphate translocase	SLC37A4 (aka G6PT1)	Neonatal	Glucose, Lactate, Triglycerides, Uric acid, Urine organic acids
Steatorrhea, Abdominal distension, Vomiting, Diarrhea	Wolman disease	Lysosomal acid lipase	LIPA	Neonatal	Cholesterol, Enzyme testing
Renal failure, Osteoporosis	Lysinuric protein intolerance	Defective cationic amino acid transport	SLC7A7	Infancy	Plasma ammonia, Serum ferritin, Urine amino acids

Table 2
Disorders with recurrent abdominal pain

Additional Distinguishing Features	Other Symptoms	Disorder and Subtype	Enzyme Defect	Gene	Age of Onset	Laboratory Testing
Flatulence, Acidic diarrhea or loose stools	Dehydration, Abdominal distension, Abdominal discomfort	Congenital sucrase-isomaltase deficiency (CSID)	Sucrase-isomaltase	*SI*	Neonatal to infancy	Duodenal or jejunal mucosal biopsy, Assay of disaccharidases
Vomiting, Poor feeding, Failure to thrive	Lethargy, Ketoacidosis, Chronic neurological problems, Hyperammonemia, Hypotonia	Ornithine transcarbamylase (OTC) deficiency	Ornithine transcarbamylase	*OTC*	Neonate, Infancy, Adolescents	Urine amino acids, Plasma amino acids, Orotic acid
		Argininosuccinic aciduria (ASA)	Argininosuccinate lyase	*ASL*	Early onset OTC typically seen in males (X-linked)	Plasma ammonia
	Ketoacidosis, Lethargy, Anorexia, Pancreatitis, Dehydration	Isovaleric aciduria (IVA)	Isovaleryl-CoA dehydrogenase	*IVD*	Infancy	Urine organic acids, Lactate, Calcium, Blood counts
		Methylmalonic aciduria (MMA)	Methylmalonyl-CoA mutase	*MMUT* aka *MCM, MUT*		
		Propionic aciduria	Propionyl-CoA carboxylase	*PCCA, PCCB*		
Neuropathy, Psychiatric symptoms	Tachycardia, Vomiting, Constipation, Diarrhea	Acute intermittent porphyria (AIP)	Hydroxymethylbilane synthase	*HMBS*	Post pubescent	Urine porphobilinogen, Urine aminolevulinic acid
		Aminolevulinic acid dehydratase deficiency	Aminolevulinic acid dehydratase	*ALAD*		Urine porphyrins, Fecal porphyrins
	Same as AIP, 20% have cutaneous photosensitivity	Hereditary coproporphyria (HCP)	Coproporphyrinogen oxidase	*CPOX*	Post pubescent	
	Same as AIP, 80% have cutaneous photosensitivity	Variegate porphyria (VP)	Protoporphyrinogen oxidase	*PPOX*	Post pubescent	
	Liver failure, Vomiting, Bleeding, Hepatomegaly	Tyrosinemia type I	Fumarylacetoacetase	*FAH*	Neonatal to infancy	Urine organic acids, Succinylacetone, Plasma amino acids, Urine aminolevulinic acid

Clinical features	Disease	Protein/Enzyme	Gene	Age of onset	Diagnostic tests
Lactic acidosis Liver disease Cardiomyopathy Hypotonia Neuropathy Retinopathy Rhabdomyolysis	Trifunctional protein deficiency Long-chain 3-hydroxyacyl-CoA dehydrogenase deficiency (LCHAD)	long-chain 3-hydroxyacyl-CoA dehydrogenase, long-chain enoyl-CoA hydratase, and long-chain thiolase Long-chain 3-hydroxyacyl-CoA dehydrogenase	*HADHA*	Late infancy – severe phenotype Adolescence to early adulthood – milder phenotype	Serum carnitine Urine carnitine Urine acylcarnitine Urine organic acids Plasma free fatty acids
Cardiomyopathy Renal tubular acidosis Vomiting Lethargy Seizures Coma	Primary carnitine deficiency Carnitine palmitoyl transferase I deficiency Medium-chain acyl-CoA dehydrogenase deficiency (MCAD)	Carnitine transporter Carnitine palmitoyl transferase I Medium-chain acyl-CoA dehydrogenase	*SLC22A5* aka *OCTN2* *CPT1A* *ACADM*	Neonate to infancy	
Pain in extremities Angiokeratomas Angiectasis Hypertrophic cardiomyopathy	Fabry disease	Alpha-galactosidase A	*GLA*	Adolescence to adult	Enzyme studies
Intestinal pseudo-obstruction Neuropathy Myopathy	MNGIE syndrome	Thymidine phosphorylase	*TYMP*	Childhood to adolescence	CSF lactate and protein Plasma thymidine and deoxyuridine
Chronic diarrhea Pyramidal tract signs Seizures Neurodevelopmental regression	Ethylmalonic encephalopathy	Mitochondrial matrix protein	*ETHE1*	Infancy	Urine organic acids Plasma acylcarnitine

propionic acidemias inhibit the first step of the urea cycle, leading to secondary hyper-ammonemia.[4,8–10] Likewise, increased ammonia levels may provoke vomiting in urea cycle disorders, such as ornithine transcarbamylase deficiency and argininosuccinic aciduria as the body attempts to excrete urea through the GI tract because ammonia is ineffectually cleared by the kidneys.[3] Medium-chain acyl-CoA dehydrogenase deficiency (MCADD) also may have hyperammonemia resulting in recurrent vomiting. These disorders typically have intermittent symptoms, most often triggered by infections, intercurrent illness, or periods of prolonged fasting. Vomiting leads to alkalosis, but, in cases of acidosis discovered in an infant or child with cyclic vomiting, the possibility of an underlying organic aciduria should be investigated. Cyclic vomiting is also observed in patients with mitochondrial dysfunction, including the disorder, mitochondrial encephalomyopathy, lactic acidosis, and stroke-like episodes (MELAS), where it represents the most common GI finding.[11,12] In these individuals, the episodes of vomiting are recurrent and occur with a periodicity that distinguishes them from other situations where frequent vomiting is observed.[13] This disorder is discussed in further detail later. Laboratory testing should include blood lactate, pyruvate, and ammonia levels, and urine organic acid and plasma amino acids analysis.[14]

PANCREATITIS

Hereditary pancreatitis is a genetic condition associated with recurrent episodes of acute pancreatitis. Beginning with a single occurrence in late childhood, episodes of pancreatitis can progress to multiple incidents over a 1-year time span. An acute episode may last from a few to several days, depending on the patient, and consist of bouts of abdominal pain, nausea, vomiting, and fever. Chronic pancreatitis develops in early adulthood, with abdominal pain, flatulence, and bloating. Pancreatic calcifications can also occur, and pancreatic fibrosis may develop in some individuals after years of inflammation, leading to a loss of pancreatic function and impairment of digestive enzyme production. The resulting disruption of the normal digestive process is followed by steatorrhea, weight loss, and protein and vitamin deficiencies. Additionally, these individuals tend to develop type 1 diabetes mellitus due to the decrease in insulin production by the affected pancreas.[15,16]

Although not typical, acute pancreatitis can be a complication of several IEMs in which acidosis, ketosis, vomiting, and abdominal pain are common during crises of metabolic decompensation.[17] The organic acidurias primarily associated with pancreatitis include isovaleric aciduria, propionic aciduria, methylmalonic aciduria, and β-ketothiolase deficiency. Pancreatitis also has been described in patients with glutaric aciduria type I and glutaric aciduria type II.[18–20] As expected, amylase and lipase are typically elevated when the patient is symptomatic. The pathogenesis of the pancreatitis observed in organic acidurias is unclear, although theories include mitochondrial dysfunction, cellular acidosis within the pancreatic acinar cell, and reactive oxygen species.[21–23] Carnitine palmitoyltransferase II deficiency also can present with recurrent pancreatitis.[24] Laboratory testing for suspected acute pancreatitis cases should include measurement of urine organic acids, plasma amino acids and plasma acylcarnitines to rule out an underlying organic aciduria or fatty acid oxidation defect. Disorders of oxidative phosphorylation, lipid disorders and homocystinuria due to cystathionine β-synthase deficiency also may present with pancreatitis.[14]

MITOCHONDRIAL DISORDERS

GI and hepatic symptoms may be a presenting feature for primary mitochondrial disease but are rarely seen in isolation. Typically, a mitochondrial disorder is not suspected until additional, more characteristic findings are present. There are a few mitochondrial disorders, however, in which GI and hepatic symptoms predominate. These include mitochondrial neuro-GI encephalomyopathy (MNGIE) and ethylmalonic encephalopathy. Other mitochondrial disorders also may present with similar symptoms, but they are minor in comparison to other overwhelming features.

Mitochondrial Neurogastrointestinal Encephalomyopathy

MNGIE is a rare, autosomal recessive disorder caused by mutations of the *TYMP* gene, which encodes thymidine phosphorylase.[25] In a majority of cases, GI dysmotility predominates the GI manifestations. Any portion of the GI tract can be affected, leading to a range of symptoms that include abdominal pain and cramping, dysphagia, early satiety, nausea, vomiting, bloating, and diverticula.[25–27] Cachexia often is seen, and individuals tend to be extremely thin.[9] Additional extra-GI symptoms can include ptosis, peripheral neuropathy, and ophthalmoparesis.[26,27]

The age of onset can be anywhere between 5 years and 60 years of age, although most cases present prior to 20 years old. GI symptoms have even been reported in a few patients less than 1 year of age.[27]

Laboratory investigations should include plasma lactate, cerebrospinal fluid lactate, and cerebrospinal fluid protein. Measurement of urine or plasma thymidine and deoxyuridine reveals elevations of these analytes, a pattern that is essential to the diagnosis. Thymidine phosphorylase enzyme activity is severely reduced when measured in either platelets or leukocytes.[27]

Ethylmalonic Encephalopathy

Ethylmalonic encephalopathy is a rare autosomal recessive mitochondrial disorder that presents with clinical symptoms shortly after birth. It is a multisystem disorder that affects the brain, GI tract, and peripheral vessels. Persistent diarrhea is an early symptom. Additional characteristic features are the presence of recurrent petechiae and orthostatic acrocyanosis affecting the hands and feet.[27] Laboratory investigations should include plasma lactate, urine organic acid, and plasma acylcarnitines analysis.

Mitochondrial Encephalomyopathy, Lactic Acidosis, and Stroke-Like Episodes

MELAS is a rare, mitochondrial disorder that typically presents between the ages of 2 years to 15 years. Delayed-onset cases and late-onset cases have been described, however, with onset between ages 15 years and 40 years and after 40 years of age, respectively.[27,28] The age of presentation and type and severity of clinical symptoms depend largely on the degree of mutant mitochondrial DNA heteroplasmy.

Although clinical presentation may vary between individuals, the hallmark symptom is a stroke-like episode occurring prior to 40 years of age. Cyclic vomiting is the most common GI manifestation; other GI findings may include failure to gain weight, abdominal pain, constipation, diarrhea, gastroparesis, intestinal dysmotility, and recurrent pancreatitis due to accumulation of lactic acid.[29] Other frequent features include short stature and hearing loss, with fatigue and exercise intolerance early symptoms.[27,28] Neurologic features can include autism, seizures, progressive dementia, severe migraines, peripheral neuropathy, and aphasia.[27–29]

HEPATIC MANIFESTATIONS

Liver disease or dysfunction is a clinical feature of several IEMs, as shown in **Box 1**. The type of hepatic manifestation and its degree of severity can vary and depend on multiple factors, including the affected metabolic pathway, the unique way in which

---

Box 1
Common laboratory hepatic manifestations

Elevated liver transaminases

Hypoglycemia

Hyperammonemia

Hypoalbuminemia

Decreased vitamin K

Decreased coagulation factors

Hyperbilirubinemia

---

the liver responds to injury, and the vicious cycle produced by the local and/or systemic accumulation of toxic intermediate metabolites as a result of the specific metabolic blockage. In a pathophysiologic sense, instability in various interdependent metabolic pathways, including protein degradation, ammonia detoxification, glycogen degradation, ketogenesis and ketone body degradation, fatty acid oxidation, heme biosynthesis, and metals metabolism, can produce physiologic consequences secondary to the particular defect. Along with the specific hepatic response to the metabolic aberration, these downstream consequences may lead to hepatic injury that progresses to hepatocellular damage, decreased hepatic function, cholestasis, or hepatomegaly, either alone or in combination.[30,31]

The clinical hepatic manifestations observed in IEMs depend on the extent of the liver's involvement in the affected metabolic pathway. There are 4 major hepatic manifestations, based on the type of hepatic injury: (1) cholestasis manifesting as jaundice, (2) hepatocellular damage manifesting as liver failure, (3) cirrhosis, and (4) hepatomegaly (**Table 3**).

Strictly in terms of organ involvement, IEMs can be classified into 2 categories: (1) those that produce sufficient structural damage to result in hepatic failure and/or cirrhosis with or without injury to other organs, such as cystic fibrosis and α_1-antitrypsin deficiency, and (2) those in which the actual metabolic aberration is exclusively or predominantly expressed in the liver but also results in damage to other organs, such as certain urea cycle defects and the hyperoxalurias.[32–34]

Although not without risk, liver transplantation has been successfully used as a treatment modality for various IEMs, including cystic fibrosis, α_1-antitrypsin deficiency, urea cycle defects, maple syrup urine disease, tyrosinemia, Wilson disease, and glycogen storage disease. In disorders where the metabolic derangement is limited to the liver, transplantation is much more effective in eliminating or reducing clinical symptoms; liver transplantation is less beneficial in disorders where there are major extrahepatic disease manifestations, although improvements in quality of life still can be significant.[35]

Cholestasis/Jaundice

Cholestatic liver disease manifests as jaundice and its etiology needs to be elucidated quickly to prevent further hepatic damage and systemic sequalae. Most cholestatic liver disease caused by an inherited metabolic disease produces conjugated hyperbilirubinemia with the exception of conditions where unconjugated hyperbilirubinemia is observed like Crigler-Najjar syndrome, an autosomal recessive form of UDP-glucuronyl transferase deficiency, and its milder autosomal

Table 3
Hepatic manifestations

Liver Failure Disease	Cholestasis	Cirrhosis Disease	Hepatomegaly
Barth hemoglobin	α₁-Antitrypsin deficiency	Alpers progressive infantile	Glycogen storage
Congenital disorders of glycosylation	Arginase deficiency	polydystrophy	disorders
Erythropoietic porphyria	Byler disease	α₁-Antitrypsin deficiency	Lysosomal storage
Galactosialidosis	Congenital disorders of glycosylation	Arginase deficiency	disorders
GM1 gangliosidosis	Cerebrotendinous xanthomatosis	Congenital disorders of glycosylation	
Mevalonic aciduria	Cholesterol synthesis defects	Cholesterol ester storage disease	
Mucopolysaccharidosis type VII	eg. (Smith-Lemli-Opitz-Syndrome)	Cystic fibrosis	
Niemann-Pick A and C	Citrin deficiency	Galactosemia	
Sialidosis type II	COG-7 deficiency	Gaucher disease	
Transaldolase deficiency	Cystic fibrosis	Glycogenosis type IV	
Fatty acid oxidation disorders	Galactosemia	Hemochromatosis	
Fructose-1,6-bisphosphatase deficiency	Bile acid biosynthesis disorders	Hereditary fructose intolerance	
Hereditary fructose intolerance	Long-chain-3-hydroxyacyl-CoA	Long-chain 3-hydroxyacyl-CoA	
Galactosemia	dehydrogenase deficiency	dehydrogenase deficiency	
Mitochondrial DNA depletion syndrome	Mevalonic aciduria	Peroxisomal disorders	
Neonatal hemochromatosis	Niemann-Pick disease type C	S-adenosylhomocysteine hydrolase deficiency	
Respiratory chain disorders	Peroxisomal disorders	Sitosterolemia	
Tyrosinemia type I	Tyrosinemia type 1	Transaldolase deficiency	
ACAD 9	Congenial hyperbilirubinemias	Tyrosinemia type I	
α₁-Antitrypsin deficiency		Wilson disease	
Cholesterol ester storage disease		Wolman disease	
Cystic fibrosis			
Propionic aciduria			
Methylmalonic aciduria			
Ketogenesis defects			
Pyruvate carboxylase deficiency			
S-adenosylhomocysteine hydrolase deficiency			
Urea cycle defects			
Wolman disease			
Wilson disease			

dominant form, Gilbert syndrome. Depending on the age of the patient, metabolic cholestatic liver disease needs to be teased out from among a group of nonmetabolic conditions, including, but not limited to, physiologic transient conjugated hyperbilirubinemia, neonatal immaturity, perinatal asphyxia, infectious diseases, and biliary obstruction, including biliary atresia and choledochal cyst. Cholestatic liver disease accompanied by dysmorphic features is commonly found in peroxisome biogenesis disorders, a group of defects affecting the α-oxidation and β-oxidation of very-long-chain fatty acids within the peroxisome.[36–38] In these so-called Zellweger spectrum disorders, variants in 1 of the 13 PEX genes responsible for peroxisome formation and/or the import of peroxisomal proteins have an impact on all peroxisomal functions. In patients with a neonatal or infantile presentation, jaundice and hyperbilirubinemia are typically found, with cirrhosis present when death occurs, usually within the first year of life. The early childhood presentation also includes hyperbilirubinemia, along with hepatomegaly and liver dysfunction, whereas the liver is spared in the milder forms of these disorders that present in adolescence or adulthood.[39,40] Progressive cholestatic liver disease is a common feature of bile acid biosynthesis disorders, in which the obstruction of normal bile flow and the accumulation of abnormal bile acids as a result of the metabolic block can cause hepatic damage.[41,42] In 3β-hydroxy-C27-steroid oxidoreductase deficiency, for example, liver enzymes are often not elevated until fibrosis is present later in life. Cholestatic liver disease may be the only or the main clinical manifestation in disorders, such as cystic fibrosis, tyrosinemia type I, and Niemann-Pick disease type C.[43]

Hepatocellular Damage/Liver Failure

Hepatocellular damage and consequent liver failure are the result of hepatocellular necrosis either by the accumulation of toxic intermediate metabolites (such as succinylacetone in the case of tyrosinemia type I, galactose 1-phosphate in galactosemia, or glucose-1-phosphate in hereditary fructose intolerance, to name a few); by disrupting cellular integrity, such as in Wilson disease, bile acid biosynthesis disorders, peroxisomal disorders, and cholesterol biosynthesis disorders; or through a combination of both mechanisms, as in tyrosinemia type I.[44–46]

Cirrhosis

Cirrhosis is defined as end-stage hepatocellular disease, when functional hepatocytes are replaced by connective tissue; this fibrosis is an apparent attempt by the liver to repair cellular damage. Many acquired syndromes (due to infectious diseases and environmental factors), vascular or biliary malformations, and IEMs ultimately can result in cirrhosis. Clinically speaking, age of onset is one of the most important factors to consider when evaluating cirrhosis, because it is dependent on the pathophysiology of the causative disorder. Most IEMs with hepatic manifestations progress to cirrhosis in the long term due to chronic hepatic injury and the associated local and systemic reactions resulting from it. Certain metabolic disorders, however, such as glycogenosis type IV, and to a lesser degree glycogen storage disease 1b, glycogen storage disease III, and glycogen storage disease type IX, may present with early onset of cirrhosis.[47–49] The cirrhosis may be caused by an autoimmune process or by steatosis progressing to nonalcoholic fatty liver disease; the hepatic glycogen storage diseases present with hyperlipidemia that can lead to steatosis.[47] In contrast, Wilson disease and α1-antitrypsin typically present later in life, depending on the variant, although a few early-onset cases have also been reported.

Hepatomegaly

Hepatomegaly is a common clinical finding in several forms of storage disorders. It can be either an early or only sign of a hepatic manifestation of an inborn error of storage metabolism. Depending on the pathophysiology of the disorder, hepatomegaly can be present with little or no effect on hepatic metabolic and synthetic control, like in several lysosomal storage disorders, including certain mucopolysaccharidoses, or may present with profound effect on homeostasis, like in glycogenosis.[7,50–54]

SUMMARY AND FUTURE DIRECTIONS

IEMs have many clinical manifestations, including GI manifestations. As technologies like next-generation sequencing, advanced metabolomics, and pharmacogenetics change the way patients are diagnosed and treated as part of a personalized medicine approach, there is an inherent risk of information overload with minimal clinical significance. Therefore, as the postgenomic era is entered, basic principles and basic first-tier laboratory testing still provide the major diagnostic framework for inherited metabolic disease and are useful guidelines whenever an underlying IEM enters consideration (**Table 4**). It is important to remain true to the spirit of medicine, which is taking care of a person's well-being by providing a full and complete clinical evaluation. Properly using currently available genetic offerings, however, such as pharmacogenetics testing to increase treatment efficacy and reduce adverse side effects, is a cost-effective and health-beneficial measure for all patients. For pediatric patients in particular, pharmacogenetics must take into account the effect that hepatic maturity has on drug metabolism and the differences between a pediatric and an adult patient response to treatment.[55–58] For a patient with a predominantly GI presentation, it also is important to bear in mind that although most metabolic disorders can be and are diagnosed during childhood, IEMs can have initial manifestations at any age, depending on the nature of the underlying molecular abnormality. Consequently, this category of disorders always should be considered when a patient's presenting GI symptoms cannot be explained by more common diseases, regardless of age.

Table 4
Common routine and biochemical genetics tests used in the diagnosis and follow-up of inborn errors of metabolism

Routine Laboratory Tests	Biochemical Genetics Tests	Inborn Errors of Metabolism
Blood glucose	Plasma acylcarnitines	Fatty acid oxidation disorders and organic acidurias
Blood lactate	Urine organic acids	Organic acidurias, aminoacidopathies,
Blood ammonia	Plasma amino acids	mitochondrial disorders
Blood pH	Urine/plasma	Urea cycle defects, organic acidurias,
Urine and blood	porphyrins	aminoacidopathies
ketones	Very-long-chain	Urea cycle defects, organic acidurias,
	fatty acids	aminoacidopathies
	Urine creatine panel	Fatty acid oxidation disorders and organic acidurias
	Urine purine/	Porphyrias
	pyrimidines	Peroxisomal disorders
	Serum carnitine	Creatine biosynthesis disorders
		Purine and pyrimidine disorders
		Primary carnitine deficiencies, fatty acid oxidation disorders, organic acidurias

REFERENCES

1. Petrides PE. Acute intermittent porphyria: mutation analysis and identification of gene carriers in a German kindred by PCR-DGGE analysis. Skin Pharmacol Appl Skin Physiol 1998;11(6):374–80.
2. Bonkovsky HL, Maddukuri VC, Yazici C, et al. Acute porphyrias in the USA: features of 108 subjects from porphyrias consortium. Am J Med 2014;127(12): 1233–41.
3. Benedict S, Nash T. The site of ammonia formation and the role of vomiting in ammonia elimination. J Biol Chem 1926;69:381–96.
4. Woods JS, Martin MD, Leroux BG. Validity of spot urine samples as a surrogate measure of 24-hour porphyrin excretion rates. Evaluation of diurnal variations in porphyrin, mercury, and creatinine concentrations among subjects with very low occupational mercury exposure. J Occup Environ Med 1998;40(12): 1090–101.
5. Bonilla Guerrero R, Karen K, Denise S, et al. The porphyrias. In: Sarafloglou K, editor. Pediatric endocrinology and inborn errors of metabolism. 2nd edition. New York: McGraw Hill; 2017. p. 461–77.
6. Fernandez-Lainez C, Ibarra-Gonzalez I, Belmont-Martinez L, et al. Tyrosinemia type I: clinical and biochemical analysis of patients in Mexico. Ann Hepatol 2014;13(2):265–72.
7. Hilz MJ, Arbustini E, Dagna L, et al. Non-specific gastrointestinal features: could it be Fabry disease? Dig Liver Dis 2018;50(5):429–37.
8. Tan ML, Liwanag MJ, Quak SH. Cyclical vomiting syndrome: recognition, assessment and management. World J Clin Pediatr 2014;3(3):54–8.
9. Fitzgerald M, Crushell E, Hickey C. Cyclic vomiting syndrome masking a fatal metabolic disease. Eur J Pediatr 2013;172(5):707–10.
10. Rinaldo P. Mitochondrial fatty acid oxidation disorders and cyclic vomiting syndrome. Dig Dis Sci 1999;44(8 Suppl):97S–102S.
11. El-Hattab AW, Scaglia F. Disorders of carnitine biosynthesis and transport. Mol Genet Metab 2015;116(3):107–12.
12. Moses J, Keilman A, Worley S, et al. Approach to the diagnosis and treatment of cyclic vomiting syndrome: a large single-center experience with 106 patients. Pediatr Neurol 2014;50(6):569–73.
13. Gelfand AA, Gallagher RC. Cyclic vomiting syndrome versus inborn errors of metabolism: A review with clinical recommendations. Headache 2016;56(1): 215–21.
14. Kahler S. Gastrointestinal and general abdominal symptoms. In: Hoffman GF, editor. Inherited metabolic diseases. Berlin: Springer-Verlag; 2010. p. 109–16.
15. Howes N, Lerch MM, Greenhalf W, et al. Clinical and genetic characteristics of hereditary pancreatitis in Europe. Clin Gastroenterol Hepatol 2004;2(3):252–61.
16. Rebours V, Levy P, Ruszniewski P. An overview of hereditary pancreatitis. Dig Liver Dis 2012;44(1):8–15.
17. Kahler SG, Sherwood WG, Woolf D, et al. Pancreatitis in patients with organic acidemias. J Pediatr 1994;124(2):239–43.
18. Lemire EG, Moroz S, Pollack B, et al. Acute pancreatitis in a patient with glutaric acidemia type I. J Pediatr 1996;128(4):589–90.
19. Liang WC, Tsai KB, Lai CL, et al. Riboflavin-responsive glutaric aciduria type II with recurrent pancreatitis. Pediatr Neurol 2004;31(3):218–21.
20. Coskun T, Gogus S, Akcoren Z, et al. Acute pancreatitis in a patient with glutaric acidemia type II. Turk J Pediatr 1997;39(3):379–85.

21. Mantadakis E, Chrysafis I, Tsouvala E, et al. Acute pancreatitis with rapid clinical improvement in a child with isovaleric acidemia. Case Rep Pediatr 2013;2013: 721871.

22. Bultron G, Seashore MR, Pashankar DS, et al. Recurrent acute pancreatitis associated with propionic acidemia. J Pediatr Gastroenterol Nutr 2008;47(3):370–1.

23. Niederau C, Schultz HU, Letko G. Involvement of free radicals in the pathophysiology of chronic pancreatitis: potential of treatment with antioxidant and scavenger substances. Klin Wochenschr 1991;69(21–23):1018–24.

24. Tein I, Christodoulou J, Donner E, et al. Carnitine palmitoyltransferase II deficiency: a new cause of recurrent pancreatitis. J Pediatr 1994;124(6):938–40.

25. Chapman TP, Hadley G, Fratter C, et al. Unexplained gastrointestinal symptoms: think mitochondrial disease. Dig Liver Dis 2014;46(1):1–8.

26. Garone C, Tadesse S, Hirano M. Clinical and genetic spectrum of mitochondrial neurogastrointestinal encephalomyopathy. Brain 2011;134(Pt 11):3326–32.

27. Rahman S. Gastrointestinal and hepatic manifestations of mitochondrial disorders. J Inherit Metab Dis 2013;36(4):659–73.

28. Hirano M, Ricci E, Koenigsberger MR, et al. Melas: an original case and clinical criteria for diagnosis. Neuromuscul Disord 1992;2(2):125–35.

29. Sproule DM, Kaufmann P. Mitochondrial encephalopathy, lactic acidosis, and strokelike episodes: basic concepts, clinical phenotype, and therapeutic management of MELAS syndrome. Ann N Y Acad Sci 2008;1142:133–58.

30. Camargo SM, Bockenhauer D, Kleta R. Aminoacidurias: clinical and molecular aspects. Kidney Int 2008;73(8):918–25.

31. Saudubray JM, Nassogne MC, de Lonlay P, et al. Clinical approach to inherited metabolic disorders in neonates: an overview. Semin Neonatol 2002;7(1):3–15.

32. Hansen K, Horslen S. Metabolic liver disease in children. Liver Transpl 2008; 14(4):391–411.

33. Hulton SA. The primary hyperoxalurias: a practical approach to diagnosis and treatment. Int J Surg 2016;36(Pt D):649–54.

34. Greene DN, Elliott-Jelf MC, Straseski JA, et al. Facilitating the laboratory diagnosis of alpha1-antitrypsin deficiency. Am J Clin Pathol 2013;139(2):184–91.

35. Oishi K, Arnon R, Wasserstein MP, et al. Liver transplantation for pediatric inherited metabolic disorders: considerations for indications, complications, and perioperative management. Pediatr Transplant 2016;20(6):756–69.

36. Grayer J. Recognition of Zellweger syndrome in infancy. Adv Neonatal Care 2005;5(1):5–13.

37. Berendse K, Engelen M, Ferdinandusse S, et al. Zellweger spectrum disorders: clinical manifestations in patients surviving into adulthood. J Inherit Metab Dis 2016;39(1):93–106.

38. Rosewich H, Waterham H, Poll-The BT, et al. Clinical utility gene card for: Zellweger syndrome spectrum. Eur J Hum Genet 2015;23(8).

39. Baes M, Van Veldhoven PP. Hepatic dysfunction in peroxisomal disorders. Biochim Biophys Acta 2016;1863(5):956–70.

40. Klouwer FC, Berendse K, Ferdinandusse S, et al. Zellweger spectrum disorders: clinical overview and management approach. Orphanet J Rare Dis 2015;10:151.

41. Clayton PT. Disorders of bile acid synthesis. J Inherit Metab Dis 2011;34(3): 593–604.

42. Heubi JE, Setchell KDR, Bove KE. Inborn errors of bile acid metabolism. Clin Liver Dis 2018;22(4):671–87.

43. Amiri M, Kuech EM, Shammas H, et al. The pathobiochemistry of gastrointestinal symptoms in a patient with niemann-pick type C disease. JIMD Rep 2016;25: 25–9.
44. Segal S, Wehrli S, Yager C, et al. Pathways of galactose metabolism by galactosemics: evidence for galactose conversion to hepatic UDPglucose. Mol Genet Metab 2006;87(2):92–101.
45. Jankowska I, Socha P. Progressive familial intrahepatic cholestasis and inborn errors of bile acid synthesis. Clin Res Hepatol Gastroenterol 2012;36(3):271–4.
46. Chanprasert S, Scaglia F. Adult liver disorders caused by inborn errors of metabolism: review and update. Mol Genet Metab 2015;114(1):1–10.
47. Baertling F, Mayatepek E, Gerner P, et al. Liver cirrhosis in glycogen storage disease Ib. Mol Genet Metab 2013;108(3):198–200.
48. Bao Y, Kishnani P, Wu JY, et al. Hepatic and neuromuscular forms of glycogen storage disease type IV caused by mutations in the same glycogen-branching enzyme gene. J Clin Invest 1996;97(4):941–8.
49. Chen Y. 8th edition. Glycogen storage diseases, vol. 1. New York: McGraw-Hill; 2001.
50. Banikazemi M, Ullman T, Desnick RJ. Gastrointestinal manifestations of Fabry disease: clinical response to enzyme replacement therapy. Mol Genet Metab 2005; 85(4):255–9.
51. Staretz-Chacham O, Lang TC, LaMarca ME, et al. Lysosomal storage disorders in the newborn. Pediatrics 2009;123(4):1191–207.
52. Winchester B. Lysosomal diseases: diagnostic update. J Inherit Metab Dis 2014; 37(4):599–608.
53. Valayannopoulos V, Mengel E, Brassier A, et al. Lysosomal acid lipase deficiency: Expanding differential diagnosis. Mol Genet Metab 2017;120(1–2):62–6.
54. Burda P, Hochuli M. Hepatic glycogen storage disorders: what have we learned in recent years? Curr Opin Clin Nutr Metab Care 2015;18(4):415–21.
55. de Graaff LC, van Schaik RH, van Gelder T. A clinical approach to pharmacogenetics. Neth J Med 2013;71(3):145–52.
56. Bakhouche H, Slanar O. Pharmacogenetics in clinical practice. Prague Med Rep 2012;113(4):251–61.
57. Chalkidou K, Rawlins M. Pharmacogenetics and cost-effectiveness analysis: a two-way street. Drug Discov Today 2011;16(19–20):873–7.
58. Evans WE. A journey from pediatric pharmacokinetics to pharmacogenomics. J Pediatr Pharmacol Ther 2005;10(1):8–13.

Primary Immunodeficiency and the Gut

David Schwimmer, MD[a], Sarah Glover, DO[b],*

KEYWORDS

- Primary immunodeficiency disease • GI symptoms • PIDD
- Common variable immunodeficiency

KEY POINTS

- Patients with primary immunodeficiency diseases often present with gastrointestinal manifestations including chronic and recurrent diarrhea, weight loss, failure to thrive, and abdominal pain.
- Gastrointestinal symptoms in these patients may be a consequence of infection, inflammation, autoimmunity, or malignancy.
- This chapter presents the most common gastrointestinal, hepatic, and pancreatic manifestations of the primary immunodeficiency diseases, including the appropriate laboratory testing, endoscopic evaluation, and recommendations for further management.

Primary immunodeficiency diseases (PIDDs) include a group of heterogeneous disorders with immune system abnormalities characterized by various combinations of recurrent infections, autoimmunity, lymphoproliferation, granulomatous process, atopy, and malignancy.[1]

To date, more than 350 distinct PIDDs have been described by the International Union of Immunological Societies, and, although respiratory symptoms seem the most common manifestation of disease, the gastrointestinal (GI) system (including the liver, biliary tree, and pancreas) is the second most common site for complications. In total, approximately one-third of the PIDDs described in the most recent Committee Report on Inborn Errors of Immunity have some GI component or symptom involved.[2,3] In studies of patient populations, the range of PIDD patients affected by GI disease can vary from 5% to 50% and depends on the specific immune defect(s) in each patient.[4] Nevertheless, the manifestation of GI symptoms varies, not only from 1 immunodeficiency disease to another but also from patient to patient, even those with the same diagnosis.

The GI tract is the largest lymphoid organ in the body and, thus, particularly vulnerable to states of immunodeficiency. Given the near constant exposure of the

Disclosure Statement: The authors have no financial interests to disclose.
[a] UF Health, PO Box 100214, Gainesville, FL 32610, USA; [b] UF Health, PO Box 103643, Gainesville, FL 32610, USA
* Corresponding author. PO Box 100214, Gainesville, FL 32610.
E-mail address: sarah.glover@medicine.ufl.edu

immunogenic intestine to foreign antigens from viruses, bacteria, parasites, and dietary proteins, proper functioning depends on the intestinal immune system's ability to maintain homeostasis between active immunity and tolerance.[5] In the setting of dysfunction or dysregulation, as often occurs PIDDs, there arises the risk of recurrent infection, inflammation, autoimmunity, and neoplasm or malignancy.[6,7]

PIDD patients often present to their physicians with a history of infections involving the upper and lower respiratory tracts, but it is not unusual for GI symptoms and pathology to be the inciting or initial sign of an underlying immune defect.[8–10] These patients often attest to recurrent/chronic abdominal pain, diarrhea, malabsorption, and failure to thrive. Less common presentations include bloody diarrhea, abnormal liver function tests, intestinal obstruction, or pancreatic insufficiency. Given the implications associated with the diagnosis of most PIDDs as well as the significant improvement in quality of life associated with treatment, it is worthwhile for health care professionals to familiarize themselves with the diagnosis and management of these disorders.[11]

This article presents the most common GI, hepatic, and pancreatic manifestations of the PIDDs, including the appropriate laboratory testing, endoscopic evaluation, and recommendations for further management.

INFECTIOUS COMPLICATIONS

Recurrence of infectious disease is the best recognized characteristic of PIDDs. It has been recommended that any patient with severe infections from typically minimally deleterious pathogens, recurrent infections, or infection by an opportunistic microorganism be investigated for a PIDD after ruling out the possibility of HIV coinfection.[12]

Due to the different mechanisms by which the immune system responds to various classes of microorganisms, much information can be inferred by the types of microorganisms involved as well as the organ systems affected. Traditionally, B-cell predominant defects (ie, selective IgA deficiency, common variable immunodeficiency [CVID], and X-linked agammaglobulinemia [XLA]) are characterized by infections with bacterial organisms and parasites;T-cell defects (ie, immunodeficiency, polyendocrinopathy enteropathy X-linked [IPEX] syndrome) with viral and fungal infections; both B-cell and T-cell defects—combined immunodeficiency (ie, hyper-IgM syndrome, severe combined immunodeficiency [SCID], and nuclear factor [NF]-κB essential modulator [NEMO] deficiency) with viral, bacterial (including intracellular), and fungal organisms; and disorders of impaired phagocytosis (ie, chronic granulomatous disease [CGD]) with bacterial and fungal organisms.[12]

After the respiratory tract, the GI tract is the second most common site of infection in patients with PIDD. Patients may present with acute, chronic, or recurrent infections causing diarrhea, malabsorption, failure to thrive, cholangitis, or abscesses of the liver.

Infectious Diarrhea

In patients with predominant defects in humoral immunity, including those with selective IgA deficiency, CVID, and XLA, the most common identifiable cause for chronic/recurrent infectious diarrhea is infection by *Giardia lamblia*.[13–16]

G lamblia cysts are transmitted by fecal-oral means and lead to the production of trophozoites that colonize the small intestine with resultant bloating, cramping, excessive flatus, and watery diarrhea. Chronic infection, as often occurs in patients with PIDD, can cause permanent mucosal damage leading to malnutrition with vitamin deficiency, steatorrhea, and failure to thrive.[17,18] In the past, a diagnosis of giardiasis had been made by microscopic evaluation of the stool looking for cysts or trophozoites. If this initial test is inconclusive and the suspicion for infection remained high, a direct examination of duodenal aspirates by string test or endoscopic biopsy could then be attempted to yield more conclusive results.[19]

The recent introduction of stool multiplex tandem (MT) polymerase chain reaction (PCR) assays has led to the ability to detect parasitic, viral, and bacterial causes of infection with exquisite sensitivity and specificity.[20,21] MT-PCR amplifies multiple targets using an array of primer pairs but only for a limited number of cycles; samples are then divided into aliquots and each aliquot amplified with a nested pair of amplicons targeting a specie of interest. In a study comparing the sensitivity and specificity of MT-PCR, real-time PCR (RT-PCR), and conventional microscopic techniques in the detection of fecal protozoa, MT-PCR and RT-PCR correlated in 100% of cases, whereas the sensitivity of microscopy ranged from 38% to 56%.[20] Furthermore, PCR assays are reliable for proving successful eradication of infection approximately 1 week after treatment.[22] In patients with PIDD, especially those with B-cell deficiency, *Giardia* infection often persists despite appropriate treatment. For such cases, a longer course of the initial therapy regimen, the introduction of a combined regimen or a switch to a different antimicrobial class may be considered.[23,24]

Other causes of infectious diarrhea in patients with PIDD can range from common enteric organisms to those not typically associated with intestinal infection. **Table 1** provides a list of the common organisms in patients with immunodeficiency syndromes presenting with GI complaints. The management and diagnosis of prolonged diarrhea in these patients should follow a stepwise algorithm, so as to quickly rule out, identify, and treat infection while considering possible alternative causes for diarrhea. Initial evaluation with stool-based PCR testing for bacterial, viral, and parasitic organisms provides a fairly comprehensive and accurate assessment of current infection status and can provide direction regarding treatment.[25] Physicians should maintain a high suspicion for small intestinal bacterial overgrowth in PIDD patients, especially those with hypogammaglobulinemia.[26] Patients may present with chronic diarrhea and malabsorption; diagnosis can be made with hydrogen breath testing or a therapeutic trial of nonabsorbed broad-spectrum antibiotics[27,28] (see **Table 1**).

AUTOIMMUNE AND INFLAMMATORY INTESTINAL DISEASE

Chronic immune dysregulation in primary immunodeficiency often results in the development of inappropriate immune responses that can lead to autoimmunity or uncontrolled inflammation. Several studies have shown autoimmune manifestations are the second most common clinical consequence of PIDDs after infection.[29–31] Within the GI tract, liver, and biliary system, autoimmunity and inflammation in PIDDs have similar clinical manifestations as diseases seen in immunocompetent patients. Common presentations of inflammation and autoimmunity include celiac and celiac-like disease, inflammatory bowel disease (IBD) and IBD-like disease, autoimmune enteropathy, pernicious anemia and gastritis, and autoimmune liver disease.[3,18,29]

Celiac and Celiac-like Disease

Celiac disease, or celiac sprue, is a common autoimmune disorder cause by an inappropriate immune response directed against gluten, which is a protein derived from wheat, barley, and rye. Ingestion of gluten containing foods promotes an inflammatory reaction, typically within the upper small intestine, characterized by mucosal inflammation and villous atrophy.[32] Patients typically present with complaints of bloating, diarrhea, weight loss, and malabsorption. Celiac and celiac-like conditions are commonly seen in patients with selective IgA deficiency and CVID.[30,33] In

Table 1
Immunodeficiency syndromes presenting with gastrointestinal symptoms

Disease	Gastrointestinal/Liver Symptoms	Common Organisms	Inflammatory Disease	Pertinent Pathology and Notes
Predominantly antibody deficiencies				
Selective IgA deficiency[13,30,102]	Diarrhea	*G lamblia*	Increased risk for celiac disease, IBD	
CVID[14,28,38,41,112]	Chronic diarrhea, malabsorption, weight loss, hepatitis, liver dysfunction, small intestinal bacterial overgrowth	Giardia, Cryptosporidium, CMV, Salmonella, Campylobacter, Norovirus (may be related to enteropathy), *Helicobacter pylori*	Stomach: atrophic gastritis, pernicious anemia Small and large intestines: celiac-like disease, IBD-like disease, CVID enteropathy Liver/biliary: granulomatous liver disease, NRH	Celiac-like disease: villous atrophy, HLA-DQ2/DQ8 negative, unresponsive to gluten-free diet CVID enteropathy: graft-versus-host-like lesions, neutrophil infiltrates, absence of interstitial plasma cells
XLA[4,16,113]	Chronic diarrhea, malabsorption, failure to thrive, small intestinal bacterial overgrowth	Giardia, Salmonella, Campylobacter, Cryptosporidium, mycoplasma, enterovirus, coxsackievirus	IBD-like disease (with strictures and fistulas)	Unlike CD, strictures and fissures have no granulomas or plasma cells. There are no germinal centers or gut-associated lymphoid tissues
Hyperimmunoglobulin M syndromes[18,53,55,108]	Acute and chronic diarrhea, failure to thrive, oral ulcers, rectal ulcers, splenomegaly, progressive liver disease	Cryptosporidium, Giardia, Salmonella, *Entamoeba histolytica*	Sclerosing cholangitis (can progress to cirrhosis and cancer), IBD-like disease	

Combined immunodeficiencies

SCID and other combined defects involving both T cells and B cells (CD3 deficiency, adenosine deaminase (ADA) deficiency)[7,18]	Intractable diarrhea, failure to thrive, viral and opportunistic infections	Rotavirus, CMV, adenovirus, Candida	IBD-like disease, celiac-like disease, AIH	
Anhidrotic ectodermal dysplasia with immunodeficiency (NEMO deficiency)[2,114,115]	Chronic diarrhea, failure to thrive	Adenovirus, CMV, Salmonella, Candida (mucocutaneous)	May present with early-onset IBD	
Defects of phagocytes				
CGD (X-linked, autosomal recessive)[28,51,116–119]	Diarrhea, steatorrhea, protein-losing enteropathy malabsorption, failure to thrive, dysphagia, constipation, obstruction, perirectal abscess, hepatic abscess, cholecystitis	Catalase-positive organisms: Staphylococcus aureus, Burkholderia cepacia, Serratia, Chromobacterium violaceum, Nocardia, Aspergillosis, mycobacterium, Cryptococcus	Esophagus: dysmotility, spasm, ulceration Stomach: gastric outlet obstruction, eosinophilic gastritis Small and large intestine: Granulomatous enteritis and colitis (IBD-like disease with fissures and rectal abscesses) Liver: liver abscess, granulomatous hepatitis	Biopsy with microgranulomas, lack of neutrophils, increased eosinophils and pigment-laden macrophages in lamina propria Hepatic abscess usually involving Staphylococcus aureus or Pseudomonas aeruginosa
Shwachman-Diamond syndrome[7,91]	Diarrhea, steatorrhea, malabsorption		Pancreatic exocrine insufficiency	

(continued on next page)

Table 1
(continued)

Disease	Gastrointestinal/Liver Symptoms	Common Organisms	Inflammatory Disease	Pertinent Pathology and Notes
Diseases of immune dysregulation				
APECED or autoimmune polyendocrine syndrome type 1 (APS-1)[79,80,90,120,121]	Dysphagia, chronic diarrhea, malabsorption, failure to thrive, hepatitis	Candida (mucocutaneous)	Esophagus: Candida infection; Stomach: pernicious anemia, autoimmune gastritis; Intestine: celiac disease, infectious diarrhea, autoimmune enteropathy (IBD-like); Liver: AIH	
IPEX syndrome[46,120,122–124]	Bloody and nonbloody diarrhea, malnutrition, failure to thrive	*Staphylococcus, enterococcus* species, CMV, Candida	Early-onset IBD-like disease	Small bowel biopsy with villous blunting and inflammatory infiltrate
IPEX-like disease • ITCH deficiency • CD25 deficiency[81,125,126]	Chronic diarrhea within the first year of life, hepatosplenomegaly, ITCH associated with hepatitis	CD25 deficiency: recurrent CMV, Candida (esophagitis), Epstein-Barr virus infection	Early-onset IBD-like disease ITCH with AIH	Small bowel biopsy with villous blunting and inflammatory infiltrate (ITCH with lymphocytes)
IL-10 and IL-10 receptor deficiency[3,127,128]	Very-early-onset diarrhea		Very-early-onset IBD (<6 mo), usually colitis with enterocutaneous and rectovaginal fistulas	Ulcers of the intestinal mucosa with inflammatory infiltrates of the epithelium and abscesses

immunocompetent patients, a diagnosis of celiac disease can be made with above 95% confidence by checking for IgA antibodies against tissue transglutaminase.[34] Unfortunately, in patients with selective IgA deficiency, the low serum level of IgA may prevent detection by these assays. For this reason, tissue transglutaminase IgG may be a better and more accurate screening test for patients with low serum IgA.[35,36] The celiac disease common to patients with selective IgA deficiency typically responds favorably to a gluten-free diet whereas that is not the case in patients with CVID.[28,30,33,37–40] For this reason, it has been recommended that patients with CVID and villous atrophy undergo genetic haplotype testing for HLA-DQ2 and HLA-DQ8 and, only if positive, attempt a 6-month to 12-month trial of gluten-free diet with follow-up for histologic response.[28,41] Otherwise, it is suggested to treat the celiac-like disease of CVID as a separate entity from true celiac disease and proceed with treatment using short-term steroids or immunomodulators (azathioprine and 6-mercaptopurine) in addition to Ig replacement therapy.[18]

Inflammatory Bowel Disease and Inflammatory Bowel Disease–like Disease

IBD, typically subdivided into Crohn's disease (CD) and ulcerative colitis (UC), is a disorder of the GI tract characterized by chronic and recurrent inflammation. UC is characterized by continuous inflammation limited to the colon and rectum with associated bloody diarrhea and abdominal pain, whereas CD may affect any portion of the GI tract (most commonly the terminal ileum and colon) in a segmental manner and may present with abdominal pain, malnutrition, nausea, and vomiting. Histopathologically, the 2 diseases differ by the depth of bowel wall inflammation and resulting consequences: UC inflammation is limited to the intestinal mucosa with classical findings of crypt abscess on biopsy, whereas CD demonstrates transmural inflammation that may lead to fistula formation and structural changes with biopsies showing characteristic granuloma formation. The exact pathogenesis of IBD remains elusive but seems to involve multiple factors, including genetics, host immunity, the gut microbiota, and the environment.[42] Together, these factors seem to alter the state of intestinal homeostasis in patients with IBD and lead to a state of persistent inflammation.[43] It is, therefore, not surprising that in patients with immunodeficiency, and thus underlying immune dysregulation, there also is a predisposition for the manifestation of chronic intestinal inflammation.

At least 50 genetic variants associated with IBD-like intestinal inflammation have been described to date.[44] Such defects act to impair the intestinal epithelial barrier function or affect innate and adaptive immune functions, thereby resulting in an IBD-like phenotype.[2,44] Several of the more common PIDDs presenting with IBD-like disease are presented in **Tables 1** and **2**; however, a detailed discussion on the distinct monogenic forms of IBD is beyond the scope of this article and thoroughly reviewed elsewhere[44–46] (see **Table 2**).

Consistent with prior reviews, it is the authors' recommendation that in all patients presenting with very-early-onset IBD, that is, disease presenting prior to 6 years of age, or those with IBD and a consistent history of recurrent infection, failure to respond to therapy, or particularly severe disease, possible underlying PIDD be considered.[3,44,47] The authors suggest starting with endoscopic evaluation of the upper and lower GI tract (with random biopsies and terminal ileum intubation), thorough cross-sectional imaging (by either CT enterography or magnetic resonance enterography [MRE]), and ruling out underlying infection by fecal MT-PCR, *Clostridium difficile* testing, and sampling tissue for cytomegalovirus (CMV).[48–50] Endoscopy then should be followed by a basic immunologic work-up for PIDD with assessment of differential white blood cell count, evaluation of lymphocyte subsets, and immunoglobulin class

Table 2
Immune defects and laboratory testing in primary immunodeficiency diseases presenting with gastrointestinal symptoms

Disease	Immune Defect	Testing and Diagnosis	Additional Points
Selective IgA deficiency[13,30,35,102,129]	Defective maturation of B cells into IgA-secreting plasma cells	Serum IgA low or absent; normal levels of other immunoglobulins	
CVID[8,18,37,38,40,54,65,75,103]	Group of heterogeneous disorders characterized by failure of B-cell differentiation with impaired Ig secretion; T-cell abnormalities; defects in antigen-presenting cells	Marked decrease (2 SD) in serum IgG as well as a marked decrease in either IgA or IgM. Absent or poor response to protein and polysaccharide vaccines	
XLA[15,16,18,39,113]	Defect in Bruton tyrosine kinase, leading to maturation arrest of pre–B cells and failure to make mature B cells	Low to absent IgG, IgA, IgM Low to absent CD19+ B cells Absent antibody responses to vaccines and microbial antigens	
Hyperimmunoglobulin M syndromes[52,53,55,88,130,131]	X-linked (most common) defect in CD40LG gene, autosomal recessive defect in CD40	Normal or elevated IgM with low IgG, IgA, and IgE Lack of response to polysaccharide and protein vaccines	Recommend close monitoring of liver function test for signs of sclerosing cholangitis
SCID and other combined defects involving both T cells and B cells (CD3 deficiency, ADA deficiency)[3,18,132]	Decrease serum immunoglobulins Markedly diminished or absent T-cell, B-cell, and NK-cell numbers, depending on functional deficiency Diminished response to mitogens	Absent or decreased circulatory T cells Normal, increased, or decreased B cells Normal, absent, or decreased NK cells. Lack of functional antibodies Low or absent T-cell receptor excision circles on newborn screening	With the advent of newborn screening for SCID, patients are detected prior to onset of severe disease.
Anhidrotic ectodermal dysplasia with immunodeficiency (NEMO deficiency)[2,133]	X-linked (most common) due to mutation in IKBKG gene; autosomal dominant due to mutation in NFKBIA gene. Mutations impair nuclear factor-kappa-B, an essential regulator of immunity and iinflammation	Hypogammaglobulinemia, impaired vaccine response, elevated or normal IgM or IgA, reduced NK-cell cytotoxicity	Part of larger syndrome characterized by alopecia, hypohydrosis or anhydrosis, tooth anomalies

Disease	Mechanism	Immune findings	Syndrome characterization
CGD (X-linked, autosomal recessive)[18,28,58,60,117,119,134–136]	Genetic mutation (2/3 X-linked, 1/3 autosomal recessive) resulting in defective NADPH oxidase and preventing phagocyte function	Hypogammaglobulinemia Impaired neutrophil function test, usually flow cytometry dihydrorhodamine neutrophil respiratory burst assay to make diagnosis	
Shwachman-Diamond syndrome[7,91]	Mutation in Shwachman-Bodian-Diamond-syndrome (SBDS) gene, which is involved in the functioning of ribosomes, centrosome amplification, and induction of leukemia	Pancytopenia, defective neutrophil chemotaxis	Part of larger syndrome characterized by long bone abnormalities, bone marrow failure, exocrine pancreatic insufficiency Frequent complete blood cell counts, given risk of myelodysplastic syndromes or AML
Ataxia-telangiectasia[73,137,138]	Mutation in the ataxia telangiectasia, mutated (ATM) gene, leading to defect in repair of DNA double-strand breaks, oxidative stress and other genotoxic stress	Low immunoglobulin IgA, low IgG2, defective polysaccharide antibody responses, lymphopenia (especially of the naive CD4 cells)	Part of larger syndrome characterized by progressive cerebellar ataxia, telangiectasias
APECED or autoimmune polyendocrine syndrome type 1[80,139,140]	Mutation in autoimmune regulator (AIRE) gene, causing loss in central immune tolerance, leading to failure to eliminate autoreactive T cells in the thymus	Anti–tryptophan hydroxylase 1 antibodies in enteropathy	
IPEX syndrome[3,122,124,125,140]	Mutation in forkhead box P3 (FOXP3) gene, a key regulator of immune tolerance	Lack of CD4+, CD25+, FOXP3+ regulatory T cells. Eosinophilia. Serum IgE usually elevated. Anti-AIE-75 (autoimmune enteropathy-related 75 kDa antigen) antibodies in enteropathy	Syndrome characterized by enteropathy, eczema, allergy type 1 diabetes mellitus, thyroid disease, and cytopenias

(continued on next page)

Table 2
(continued)

Disease	Immune Defect	Testing and Diagnosis	Additional Points
IPEX-like syndromes[3,125]	ITCH deficiency; CD25 deficiency; STAT5b deficiency; STAT1 GOF; STAT3 GOF mutations—lead to alteration in regulatory T-cell development and function	Elevated or normal serum immunoglobulins. In all but ITCH deficiency, serum IgE normal or slightly elevated. FOXP3 present	Syndromes presenting similar to IPEX. Less cytopenias in STAT1 and ITCH
IL-10 deficiency, IL-10 R1 deficiency, IL-10 R2 deficiency[127,128,141]	Mutation in IL-10 or IL-10 receptor	Inappropriate response to functional tests using STAT3 and/or tumor necrosis factor assays	Cause of very-early-onset (<6 mo) IBD

Abbreviations: ADA, adenosine deaminase; AML, acute myelogenous leukemia; APECED, autoimmune polyendocrinopathy-candidiasis-ectodermal dystrophy; CGD, chronic granulomatous disease; CVID, combined variable immunodeficiency; GOF, gain of function; IBD, inflammatory bowel disease; IL, interleukin; IPEX, immune dysregulation, polyendocrinopathy, enteropathy and X-linked inheritance; NADPH, reduced form of nicotinamide adenine dinucleotide phosphate; NEMO, nuclear factor-kappa-B essential modulator; NK, natural killer; SCID, severe combined immunodeficiency; SD, standard deviation; STAT, signal transducer and activator of transcription; XLA, X-linked agammaglobulinemia.

and subclass quantification as well as baseline vaccine titers and postimmunization titers.[1,44,47] The results of these studies can suggest an underlying immune deficit that then may be investigated further with more detailed and specific testing under the guidance of a dedicated immunologist.[47]

LIVER, BILIARY, AND PANCREATIC INVOLVEMENT

Liver disease in PIDD, similar to luminal disease of the GI tract, may arise as a consequence of infection, inflammation, autoimmunity, malignancy, or a combination of these. In addition, many of the PIDDs may present with hepatosplenomegaly as a consequence of lymphoproliferation.[51] Multiple studies have shown that the presence of liver disease in PIDD may be associated with worse clinical outcomes. It is for this reason that patients at risk for liver involvement be checked routinely with liver function tests.[52–54]

Liver and Biliary Infections

As outlined in **Table 1**, *Cryptosporidium parvum* is the most frequently isolated pathogen in patients with GI symptoms associated with X-linked hyper-IgM syndrome. In addition to causing diarrhea, *C parvum* has been associated with biliary tree infiltration and associated cholangiopathy in several PIDDs.[53,55–57] Chronic biliary infection can be seen on liver function tests as increases in alkaline phosphatase and γ-glutamyl transferase levels. Failure to identify and treat such infection has demonstrated progression to primary sclerosing cholangitis (PSC) and cholangiocarcinoma.[56,58,59]

Patients with CGD are at increased risk for the development of persistent and recurrent hepatic abscesses.[51,58,60] Patients typically present with increased transaminases, fever, abdominal pain, fatigue, and weight loss, with cultures most commonly revealing infection due to *Staphylococcus aureus,* or less commonly, *Pseudomonas aeruginosa*.[18,61] Other reports have also demonstrated the appearance of liver abscesses in hyper-IgM syndrome[62] and hyper-IgE syndrome.[63] The management of these liver abscesses often is difficult, requiring steroids and antibiotics or surgical resection.[60,64]

For PIDD patients presenting with elevation in liver function tests, consideration must be made for underlying viral infections due to Epstein-Barr virus, CMV, and HIV.[65] A note should also be made of the vulnerability for chronic hepatitis C in adult PIDD patients who had received transfusions or immunoglobulin therapy in the early 1990s prior to the identification of hepatitis C.[66] It is, therefore, reasonable to screen all PIDD patients at risk for HCV with PCR testing and to treat with the appropriate direct-acting antiviral regimen.[67,68]

Inflammatory and Autoimmune Liver Disease

Nodular regenerative hyperplasia (NRH) is an uncommon liver disease characterized by the development of regenerative nodules through the liver in the absence of fibrosis.[69] In addition to being associated with medications and rheumatological and hematological diseases, NRH is the most common histologic finding seen in PIDD patients with liver disease.[51,70,71] Clinically, NRH may present with noncirrhotic portal hypertension, splenomegaly, cytopenias, and liver enzyme abnormalities.[72] Several studies show an increase in alkaline phosphatase as the most commonly associated liver enzyme abnormality.[51,70] Malamut and colleagues[70] described a series of 23 patients with PIDD and liver abnormalities (by laboratory tests, imaging, or evidence of portal hypertension) who had undergone liver biopsy. Among those studied, 16/19 CVID, 3/3 hyper-IgM, and 1/1 XLA patients demonstrated evidence of NRH on biopsy. NRH also has been described in patients with CGD and ataxia telangiectasia.[51,73]

Granulomatous liver disease is commonly found in patients with CGD and less commonly in those with CVID. In a series of 31 patients with liver biopsies adequate for evaluation, 23/31 had evidence of granulomata (74.2%). In another study by Ardenez and Cunningham-Rundles[74] investigating the incidence of granulomatous disease in CVID, 37/455 patients (8.1%) had evidence of granulomas affecting the lungs (54%), lymph nodes (43%), and/or liver (32%). Treatment of granulomatous lesions in CVID may include a combination of steroids, immunomodulators, or anti–tumor necrosis factor antibodies.[65,75–77]

Other autoimmune and inflammatory liver diseases seen in patients with PIDD include autoimmune hepatitis (AIH), primary biliary cholangitis (PBC), and PSC. AIH is an inflammatory liver disease typically presenting with elevated aminotransferases and is associated with a high risk of mortality if left untreated.[78] AIH has been demonstrated in patients with CGD, autoimmune polyendocrinopathy-candidiasis-ectodermal dystrophy (APECED) (or autoimmune polyendocrine syndrome type 1), ITCH deficiency (E3 ubiquitin ligase deficiency), and activation-induced cytidine deaminase deficiency.[79–83] PBC, which has been seen in a few patients with CVID, is characterized by progressive damage to the interlobular bile ducts with resultant ductopenia, cholestasis, and bile acid retention.[54,84,85] In immunocompetent patients, a diagnosis of AIH and PBC includes serum testing for autoantibodies: anti–smooth muscle antibody and anti–liver/kidney microsomal antibody type 1 for AIH and antimitochondrial antibodies for PBC.[29] As is the case with antibody testing for celiac disease in PIDD, the circulating levels of these antibodies may be low or undetectable.[29] Diagnosis, therefore, may depend on the results of biopsy specimens.[29,54,59]

In PSC, chronic inflammation of the biliary epithelium leads to chronic cholestasis and multifocal bile duct structuring, which can progress to liver fibrosis and hepatic failure.[86,87] As discussed previously, the development of PSC can result as a consequence of underlying chronic biliary infection with C parvum.[55,88] Rodrigues and colleagues,[59] in their review of 35 children with PIDD and evidence of clinical liver disease, found 21 patients (60%) had evidence of sclerosing cholangitis by imaging or histology that was not necessarily dependent on C parvum coinfection. Additionally, evidence for PSC in the absence of underlying infection has been seen in the gain-of-function (GOF) mutation of the p110δ catalytic subunit of the phosphatidylinositol-3-OH kinase, which subsequently required liver transplant.[89]

Pancreatic Exocrine Function

Few PIDDs are characterized by the presence of pancreatic dysfunction. Among these include Shwachman-Diamond syndrome, APECED, and cystic fibrosis. In all 3 conditions, pancreatic insufficiency is 1 among many complications of the underlying genetic defect.[90–92] Nevertheless, patients presenting with pancreatic exocrine insufficiency typically describe steatorrhea or diarrhea, abdominal pain, bloating, and failure to thrive. Testing for pancreatic exocrine insufficiency in such patients includes measuring serum trypsin (which also detects trypsinogen), 72-hour fecal fat collection, fecal elastase testing on solid or semisolid stool, or direct testing of pancreatic secretions by oroduodenal tube or endoscopy after secretin stimulation.[93] Diagnosis is assured when supplementation with pancreatic enzymes results in improvement in steatorrhea and resolution of malnutrition.

NODULAR LYMPHOID HYPERPLASIA AND MALIGNANCY

Nodular lymphoid hyperplasia (NLH) is a benign condition seen most commonly in patients with antibody-deficiency syndromes (except those with agammaglobulinemia). It has been described as multiple small nodules, usually 2 mm to 10 mm in diameter and usually arising in the small intestine but also seen in the stomach, colon, and rectum.[94] On imaging studies, these nodules can be easily confused with CD and require endoscopic evaluation for diagnosis.[95] It seems that most cases of NLH are discovered incidentally. Some patients present, however, with symptoms of abdominal pain, diarrhea, occult bleeding, or malabsorption, or, rarely, obstruction.[18,96] Few reports suggest NLH may be a risk factor for the development of intestinal lymphoma.[94,97,98] The development of intestinal lymphomas has been reported in other immunodeficiency syndromes even in the absence of NLH.[99]

PIDDs have long been associated with increased risk for hematologic and solid organ malignancy.[88,100,101] In a large, population-based cohort of patients with selective IgA deficiency, there was shown a small, but statistically significant, increased risk of nondescript GI cancers.[102] The most recent data from the US Immunodeficiency Network suggest that patients with CVID have a significantly increased risk for gastric cancer.[100] These findings are consistent with other population studies and reviews suggesting the atrophic gastritis, intestinal metaplasia, and pernicious anemia seen in patients with CVID eventually may develop into gastric adenocarcinoma.[18,100,103] Although patients with CVID did not show an increased risk for colon cancer, it is the authors' recommendation that patients with PIDD and established IBD-like disease undergo surveillance colonoscopy every 1 year to 2 years.[100]

Patients with PIDD, especially hyper-IgM syndrome, who develop chronic liver and biliary disease are at increased risk for the development of primary liver and biliary malignancies.[52,88,104] Given this increased risk, some groups recommend cancer screening for patients with PSC by magnetic resonance cholangiopancreatography (MRCP) and serum cancer antigen 19-9 levels every 6 months.[104]

NUTRITION

All patients with PIDD affecting the GI tract are at increased risk for malabsorption and failure to thrive. Chronic diarrhea (due to infection or inflammation), histologic changes within the intestine, pancreatic exocrine insufficiency, NLH, and recurrent infections can lead to decreased absorption, increased nutritional wasting, and overall higher metabolic demand.[105] The increased risk for malabsorption and failure to thrive was confirmed by Malamut and colleagues,[41] in their evaluation of 50 patients with CVID and GI symptoms, as biological evidence of malabsorption was seen in 54% of their cohort. Initial evaluation should include measurement of body mass index, albumin, and prealbumin levels to assess global degree of malnutrition.[93] In children, growth and weight charts should be monitored closely. The authors recommend screening for nutrient deficiency with serum testing for iron deficiency, folic acid, zinc, selenium, copper, magnesium, calcium, and vitamin D as well as vitamins A, B_{12}, E, and K.[106-110] Protein-losing enteropathy should be assessed with stool α_1-antitrypsin (especially in those patients receiving immunoglobulin therapy and those with chronic diarrhea).[107,108,111] In patients with concern for pancreatic exocrine insufficiency, pancreatic function may be screened with serum trypsin/trypsinogen and stool elastase, as discussed previously. Deficiency in a single mineral or vitamin may be managed with repletion and dietary recommendations. It is not uncommon for patients with PIDD and sustained failure to thrive to require total parenteral nutrition to sustain caloric needs.[41,54,108]

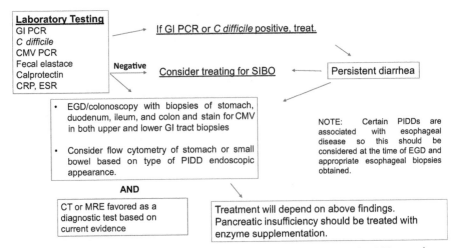

Fig. 1. Suggested evaluation of diarrhea in PIDD. CRP, C-reactive protein; EGD, esophago-gastroduodenoscopy; ESR, erythrocyte sedimentation rate; MRE, magnetic resonance enter-ography; SIBO, small intestinal bacterial overgrowth.

SUMMARY

Patients with PIDDs suffer a host of complications, ranging from infection to inflammation to autoimmunity to malignancy. Patients with GI manifestations of these diseases commonly present to their physicians with chronic diarrhea, weight loss, failure to thrive, and fatigue. The evaluation of such symptoms should progress in a stepwise manner by first ruling out underlying infection with stool studies and blood tests, followed by endoscopic evaluation (using upper endoscopy, colonoscopy, and capsule endoscopy when necessary), cross-sectional imaging (with MRI enterography), and assessment of nutritional status (**Fig. 1**). Treatment and further evaluation depend on findings and should involve coordination with a multidisciplinary team, including immunologists, nutritionists/dieticians, gastroenterologists, and infectious disease experts.

REFERENCES

1. Raje N, Dinakar C. Overview of immunodeficiency disorders. Immunol Allergy Clin 2015;35(4):599–623.
2. Picard C, Bobby Gaspar H, Al-Herz W, et al. International union of immunological societies: 2017 primary immunodeficiency diseases committee report on inborn errors of immunity. J Clin Immunol 2018;38(1):96–128.
3. Hartono S, Ippoliti MR, Mastroianni M, et al. Gastrointestinal disorders associated with primary immunodeficiency diseases. Clin Rev Allergy Immunol 2018. [Epub ahead of print].
4. Atarod L, Raissi A, Aghamohammadi A, et al. A review of gastrointestinal disorders in patients with primary antibody immunodeficiencies during a 10-year period (1990-2000), in children hospital medical center. Iran J Allergy Asthma Immunol 2003;2(2):75–9.
5. Reis BS, Mucida D. The role of the intestinal context in the generation of tolerance and inflammation. Clin Dev Immunol 2012;2012:157948.

6. Kalha I, Sellin JH. Common variable immunodeficiency and the gastrointestinal tract. Curr Gastroenterol Rep 2004;6(5):377–83.
7. Reda SM. Gastrointestinal manifestations in children with primary immunodeficiency diseases. Egypt J Pediatr Allergy Immunol 2017;15(1):3–8.
8. Pecoraro A, Nappi L, Crescenzi L, et al. Chronic diarrhea in common variable immunodeficiency: a case series and review of the literature. J Clin Immunol 2018;38(1):67–76.
9. Seymour B, Miles J, Haeney M. Primary antibody deficiency and diagnostic delay. J Clin Pathol 2005;58(5):546–7.
10. Al-Muhsen S. Gastrointestinal and hepatic manifestations of primary immune deficiency diseases. Saudi J Gastroenterol 2010;16(2):66–74.
11. Gardulf A, Nicolay U. Replacement IgG therapy and self-therapy at home improve the health-related quality of life in patients with primary antibody deficiencies. Curr Opin Allergy Clin Immunol 2006;6(6):434–42.
12. Costa-Carvalho BT, Grumach AS, Franco JL, et al. Attending to warning signs of primary immunodeficiency diseases across the range of clinical practice. J Clin Immunol 2014;34(1):10–22.
13. Yazdani R, Azizi G, Abolhassani H, et al. Selective IgA deficiency: epidemiology, pathogenesis, clinical phenotype, diagnosis, prognosis and management. Scand J Immunol 2017;85(1):3–12.
14. Oksenhendler E, Gérard L, Fieschi C, et al, DEFI Study Group. Infections in 252 patients with common variable immunodeficiency. Clin Infect Dis 2008;46(10): 1547–54.
15. Barmettler S, Otani IM, Minhas J, et al. Gastrointestinal Manifestations in X-linked Agammaglobulinemia. J Clin Immunol 2017;37(3):287–94.
16. Winkelstein JA, Marino MC, Lederman HM, et al. X-linked agammaglobulinemia: report on a United States registry of 201 patients. Medicine (Baltimore) 2006; 85(4):193–202.
17. Lengerich EJ, Addiss DG, Juranek DD. Severe giardiasis in the United States. Clin Infect Dis 1994;18(5):760–3.
18. Agarwal S, Mayer L. Diagnosis and treatment of gastrointestinal disorders in patients with primary immunodeficiency. Clin Gastroenterol Hepatol 2013;11(9): 1050–63.
19. Ortega YR, Adam RD. Giardia: overview and update. Clin Infect Dis 1997;25(3): 545–9.
20. Stark D, Al-Qassab SE, Barratt JLN, et al. Evaluation of multiplex tandem real-time PCR for detection of Cryptosporidium spp., Dientamoeba fragilis, Entamoeba histolytica, and Giardia intestinalis in Clinical Stool Samples. J Clin Microbiol 2011;49(1):257–62.
21. van Maarseveen NM, Wessels E, de Brouwer CS, et al. Diagnosis of viral gastroenteritis by simultaneous detection of Adenovirus group F, Astrovirus, Rotavirus group A, Norovirus genogroups I and II, and Sapovirus in two internally controlled multiplex real-time PCR assays. J Clin Virol 2010;49(3):205–10.
22. van den Bijllaardt W, Overdevest IT, Buiting AG, et al. Rapid clearance of Giardia lamblia DNA from the gut after successful treatment. Clin Microbiol Infect 2014;20(11):O972–4.
23. Abboud P, Lemée V, Gargala G, et al. Successful treatment of metronidazole- and albendazole-resistant giardiasis with nitazoxanide in a patient with acquired immunodeficiency syndrome. Clin Infect Dis 2001;32(12):1792–4.
24. Granados CE, Reveiz L, Uribe LG, et al. Drugs for treating giardiasis. Cochrane Database Syst Rev 2012;(12):CD007787.

25. Jex AR, Stanley KK, Lo W, et al. Detection of diarrhoeal pathogens in human faeces using an automated, robotic platform. Mol Cell Probes 2012;26(1):11–5.
26. Pignata C, Budillon G, Monaco G, et al. Jejunal bacterial overgrowth and intestinal permeability in children with immunodeficiency syndromes. Gut 1990; 31(8):879–82.
27. Rezaie A, Buresi M, Lembo A, et al. Hydrogen and methane-based breath testing in gastrointestinal disorders: the North American consensus. Am J Gastroenterol 2017;112(5):775–84.
28. Uzzan M, Ko HM, Mehandru S, et al. Gastrointestinal disorders associated with common variable immune deficiency (CVID) and chronic granulomatous disease (CGD). Curr Gastroenterol Rep 2016;18(4):17.
29. Azizi G, Ziaee V, Tavakol M, et al. Approach to the management of autoimmunity in primary immunodeficiency. Scand J Immunol 2017;85(1):13–29.
30. Ludvigsson JF, Neovius M, Hammarström L. Association between IgA deficiency & other autoimmune conditions: a population-based matched cohort study. J Clin Immunol 2014;34(4):444–51.
31. Blazina Š, Markelj G, Jeverica AK, et al. Autoimmune and inflammatory manifestations in 247 patients with primary immunodeficiency-a report from the Slovenian National Registry. J Clin Immunol 2016;36(8):764–73.
32. Green PHR, Cellier C. Celiac disease. N Engl J Med 2007;357(17):1731–43.
33. Jørgensen SF, Reims HM, Frydenlund D, et al. A cross-sectional study of the prevalence of gastrointestinal symptoms and pathology in patients with common variable immunodeficiency. Am J Gastroenterol 2016;111(10):1467–75.
34. Hill ID. What are the sensitivity and specificity of serologic tests for celiac disease? Do sensitivity and specificity vary in different populations? Gastroenterology 2005;128(4 Suppl 1):S25–32.
35. Prince HE, Norman GL, Binder WL. Immunoglobulin A (IgA) deficiency and alternative celiac disease-associated antibodies in sera submitted to a reference laboratory for endomysial IgA testing. Clin Diagn Lab Immunol 2000; 7(2):192–6.
36. Dahlbom I, Olsson M, Forooz NK, et al. Immunoglobulin G (IgG) anti-tissue transglutaminase antibodies used as markers for IgA-deficient celiac disease patients. Clin Diagn Lab Immunol 2005;12(2):254–8.
37. Baldovino S, Montin D, Martino S, et al. Common variable immunodeficiency: crossroads between infections, inflammation and autoimmunity. Autoimmun Rev 2013;12(8):796–801.
38. Daniels JA, Lederman HM, Maitra A, et al. Gastrointestinal tract pathology in patients with common variable immunodeficiency (CVID): a clinicopathologic study and review. Am J Surg Pathol 2007;31(12):1800–12.
39. Washington K, Stenzel TT, Buckley RH, et al. Gastrointestinal pathology in patients with common variable immunodeficiency and X-linked agammaglobulinemia. Am J Surg Pathol 1996;20(10):1240–52.
40. Cunningham-Rundles C. The many faces of common variable immunodeficiency. Hematol Am Soc Hematol Educ Program 2012;2012(1):301–5.
41. Malamut G, Verkarre V, Suarez F, et al. The enteropathy associated with common variable immunodeficiency: the delineated frontiers with celiac disease. Am J Gastroenterol 2010;105(10):2262–75.
42. Cosnes J, Gower–Rousseau C, Seksik P, et al. Epidemiology and natural history of inflammatory bowel diseases. Gastroenterology 2011;140(6):1785–94.e4.
43. Atreya R, Neurath MF. IBD pathogenesis in 2014:Molecular pathways controlling barrier function in IBD. Nat Rev Gastroenterol Hepatol 2015;12:67–8.

44. Uhlig HH, Schwerd T, Koletzko S, et al. The diagnostic approach to monogenic very early onset inflammatory bowel disease. Gastroenterology 2014;147(5): 990–1007.e3.
45. Uhlig HH. Monogenic diseases associated with intestinal inflammation: implications for the understanding of inflammatory bowel disease. Gut 2013;62(12): 1795–805.
46. Uhlig HH, Schwerd T. From genes to mechanisms: the expanding spectrum of monogenic disorders associated with inflammatory bowel disease. Inflamm Bowel Dis 2016;22(1):202–12.
47. Tegtmeyer D, Seidl M, Gerner P, et al. Inflammatory bowel disease caused by primary immunodeficiencies—Clinical presentations, review of literature, and proposal of a rational diagnostic algorithm. Pediatr Allergy Immunol 2017; 28(5):412–29.
48. Levine A, Griffiths A, Markowitz J, et al. Pediatric modification of the Montreal classification for inflammatory bowel disease: the Paris classification. Inflamm Bowel Dis 2011;17(6):1314–21.
49. Chalian M, Ozturk A, Oliva-Hemker M, et al. MR enterography findings of inflammatory bowel disease in pediatric patients. Am J Roentgenol 2011;196(6): W810–6.
50. Turner D, Travis SPL, Griffiths AM, et al, European Crohn's and Colitis Organization, Porto IBD Working Group, European Society of Pediatric Gastroenterology, Hepatology, and Nutrition. Consensus for managing acute severe ulcerative colitis in children: a systematic review and joint statement from ECCO, ESPGHAN, and the Porto IBD Working Group of ESPGHAN. Am J Gastroenterol 2011; 106(4):574–88.
51. Hussain N, Feld JJ, Kleiner DE, et al. Hepatic abnormalities in patients with chronic granulomatous disease. Hepatology 2007;45(3):675–83.
52. de la Morena MT, Leonard D, Torgerson TR, et al. Long-term outcomes of 176 patients with X-linked hyper-IgM syndrome treated with or without hematopoietic cell transplantation. J Allergy Clin Immunol 2017;139(4):1282–92.
53. Levy J, Espanol-Boren T, Thomas C, et al. Clinical spectrum of X-linked hyper-IgM syndrome. J Pediatr 1997;131(1 Pt 1):47–54.
54. Cunningham-Rundles C, Bodian C. Common variable immunodeficiency: clinical and immunological features of 248 patients. Clin Immunol 1999;92(1): 34–48.
55. Winkelstein JA, Marino MC, Ochs H, et al. The X-linked hyper-IgM syndrome: clinical and immunologic features of 79 patients. Medicine (Baltimore) 2003; 82(6):373–84.
56. Kotlarz D, Ziętara N, Uzel G, et al. Loss-of-function mutations in the IL-21 receptor gene cause a primary immunodeficiency syndrome. J Exp Med 2013;210(3): 433–43.
57. Hadzic N, Heaton ND, Francavilla R, et al. Paediatric sclerosing cholangitis associated with primary immunodeficiencies. J Pediatr Gastroenterol Nutr 1999;28(5):579.
58. Winkelstein JA, Marino MC, Johnston RB, et al. Chronic granulomatous disease. Report on a national registry of 368 patients. Medicine (Baltimore) 2000;79(3): 155–69.
59. Rodrigues F, Davies EG, Harrison P, et al. Liver disease in children with primary immunodeficiencies. J Pediatr 2004;145(3):333–9.
60. Lublin M, Bartlett DL, Danforth DN, et al. Hepatic abscess in patients with chronic granulomatous disease. Ann Surg 2002;235(3):383–91.

61. Bennett N, Maglione PJ, Wright BL, et al. Infectious complications in patients with chronic granulomatous disease. J Pediatric Infect Dis Soc 2018; 7(suppl_1):S12–7.

62. Shah I, Rahangdale A, Bhatnagar S. Liver abscesses and hyper IgM syndrome. J Fam Med Prim Care 2013;2(2):206–8.

63. Nandy S, Shah I. Liver abscess in a boy with hyper IgE syndrome. J Fam Med Prim Care 2016;5(2):491–2.

64. Leiding JW, Freeman AF, Marciano BE, et al. Corticosteroid therapy for liver abscess in chronic granulomatous disease. Clin Infect Dis 2012;54(5):694–700.

65. Song J, Lleo A, Yang GX, et al. Common variable immunodeficiency and liver involvement. Clin Rev Allergy Immunol 2018;55(3):340–51.

66. Razvi S, Schneider L, Jonas MM, et al. Outcome of intravenous immunoglobulin-transmitted hepatitis C virus infection in primary immunodeficiency. Clin Immunol 2001;101(3):284–8.

67. World Health Organization, Thomson E, Selvapatt N. Guidelines for the screening care and treatment of persons with chronic hepatitis C infection: updated version. In: Malhotra B, editor. Geneva: World Health Organization; 2016. p. 140.

68. Ruffner MA, Sullivan KE, Henrickson SE. Recurrent and Sustained Viral Infections in Primary Immunodeficiencies. Front Immunol 2017;8:665.

69. Reshamwala PA, Kleiner DE, Heller T. Nodular regenerative hyperplasia: Not all nodules are created equal. Hepatology 2006;44(1):7–14.

70. Malamut G, Ziol M, Suarez F, et al. Nodular regenerative hyperplasia: The main liver disease in patients with primary hypogammaglobulinemia and hepatic abnormalities. J Hepatol 2008;48(1):74–82.

71. Ward C, Lucas M, Piris J, et al. Abnormal liver function in common variable immunodeficiency disorders due to nodular regenerative hyperplasia. Clin Exp Immunol 2008;153(3):331–7.

72. Khanna R, Sarin SK. Non-cirrhotic portal hypertension – diagnosis and management. J Hepatol 2014;60(2):421–41.

73. Milligan KL, Schirm K, Leonard S, et al. Ataxia telangiectasia associated with nodular regenerative hyperplasia. J Clin Immunol 2016;36(8):739–42.

74. Ardeniz Ö, Cunningham-Rundles C. Granulomatous disease in common variable immunodeficiency. Clin Immunol 2009;133(2):198–207.

75. Boursiquot JN, Gérard L, Malphettes M, et al. Granulomatous disease in CVID: retrospective analysis of clinical characteristics and treatment efficacy in a cohort of 59 patients. J Clin Immunol 2013;33(1):84–95.

76. Thatayatikom A, Thatayatikom S, White AJ. Infliximab treatment for severe granulomatous disease in common variable immunodeficiency: a case report and review of the literature. Ann Allergy Asthma Immunol 2005;95(3):293–300.

77. Franxman TJ, Howe LE, Baker JR Jr. Infliximab for treatment of granulomatous disease in patients with common variable immunodeficiency. J Clin Immunol 2014;34(7):820–7.

78. Hennes EM, Zeniya M, Czaja AJ, et al, International Autoimmune Hepatitis Group. Simplified criteria for the diagnosis of autoimmune hepatitis. Hepatology 2008;48(1):169–76.

79. Obermayer-Straub P, Perheentupa J, Braun S, et al. Hepatic autoantigens in patients with autoimmune polyendocrinopathy-candidiasis-ectodermal dystrophy. Gastroenterology 2001;121(3):668–77.

80. Kluger N, Jokinen M, Krohn K, et al. Gastrointestinal manifestations in APECED syndrome. J Clin Gastroenterol 2013;47(2):112–20.

81. Lohr NJ, Molleston JP, Strauss KA, et al. Human ITCH E3 ubiquitin ligase deficiency causes syndromic multisystem autoimmune disease. Am J Hum Genet 2010;86(3):447–53.

82. Durandy A, Cantaert T, Kracker S, et al. Potential roles of activation-induced cytidine deaminase in promotion or prevention of autoimmunity in humans. Autoimmunity 2013;46(2):148–56.

83. Gargouri L, Safi F, Mejdoub I, et al. Auto-immune hepatitis in chronic granulomatous disease in a 2-year-old girl. Arch Pediatr 2015;22(5):518–22 [in French].

84. Invernizzi P, Floreani A, Carbone M, et al. Primary biliary cholangitis: advances in management and treatment of the disease. Dig Liver Dis 2017;49(8):841–6.

85. Xiao X, Miao Q, Chang C, et al. Common variable immunodeficiency and autoimmunity – an inconvenient truth. Autoimmun Rev 2014;13(8):858–64.

86. Singh S, Talwalkar JA. Primary sclerosing cholangitis: diagnosis, prognosis, and management. Clin Gastroenterol Hepatol 2013;11(8):898–907.

87. Mahdavinia M, Mirsaeidi M, Bishehsari F, et al. Primary sclerosing cholangitis in common variable immune deficiency. Allergol Int 2015;64(2):187–9.

88. Hayward AR, Levy J, Facchetti F, et al. Cholangiopathy and tumors of the pancreas, liver, and biliary tree in boys with X-linked immunodeficiency with hyper-IgM. J Immunol 1997;158(2):977–83.

89. Hartman HN, Niemela J, Hintermeyer MK, et al. Gain of function mutations of PIK3CD as a cause of primary sclerosing cholangitis. J Clin Immunol 2015; 35(1):11–4.

90. Perheentupa J. APS-I/APECED: the clinical disease and therapy. Endocrinol Metab Clin 2002;31(2):295–320.

91. Myers KC, Bolyard AA, Otto B, et al. Variable clinical presentation of shwachman-diamond syndrome: update from the North-American shwachman-diamond syndrome registry. J Pediatr 2014;164(4):866–70.

92. Gibson-Corley KN, Meyerholz DK, Engelhardt JF. Pancreatic pathophysiology in cystic fibrosis. J Pathol 2016;238(2):311–20.

93. Forsmark CE. Diagnosis and management of exocrine pancreatic insufficiency. Curr Treat Options Gastroenterol 2018;16(3):306–15.

94. Albuquerque A. Nodular lymphoid hyperplasia in the gastrointestinal tract in adult patients: a review. World J Gastrointest Endosc 2014;6(11):534–40.

95. Plumb AA, Pendsé DA, McCartney S, et al. Lymphoid nodular hyperplasia of the terminal ileum can mimic active Crohn's disease on MR enterography. Am J Roentgenol 2014;203(4):W400–7.

96. Garg V, Lipka S, Rizvon K, et al. Diffuse nodular lymphoid hyperplasia of intestine in selective IgG 2 subclass deficiency, autoimmune thyroiditis, and autoimmune hemolytic anemia: case report and literature review. J Gastrointestin Liver Dis 2012;21(4):431–4.

97. Chiaramonte C, Glick SN. Nodular lymphoid hyperplasia of the small bowel complicated by jejunal lymphoma in a patient with common variable immune deficiency syndrome. AJR Am J Roentgenol 1994;163(5):1118–9.

98. Castellano G, Moreno D, Galvao O, et al. Malignant lymphoma of jejunum with common variable hypogammaglobulinemia and diffuse nodular hyperplasia of the small intestine. A case study and literature review. J Clin Gastroenterol 1992;15(2):128–35.

99. Lucas KG, Ungar D, Comito M, et al. Epstein Barr virus induced lymphoma in a child with IPEX syndrome. Pediatr Blood Cancer 2008;50(5):1056–7.

100. Mayor PC, Eng KH, Singel KL, et al. Cancer in primary immunodeficiency diseases: cancer incidence in the United States immune deficiency network registry. J Allergy Clin Immunol 2018;141(3):1028–35.
101. Gathmann B, Mahlaoui N, CEREDIH, et al. Clinical picture and treatment of 2212 patients with common variable immunodeficiency. J Allergy Clin Immunol 2014; 134(1):116–26.
102. Ludvigsson JF, Neovius M, Ye W, et al. IgA deficiency and risk of cancer: a population-based matched cohort study. J Clin Immunol 2015;35(2):182–8.
103. Leone P, Vacca A, Dammacco F, et al. Common variable immunodeficiency and gastric malignancies. Int J Mol Sci 2018;19(2) [pii:E451].
104. Khaderi SA, Sussman NL. Screening for malignancy in primary sclerosing cholangitis (PSC). Curr Gastroenterol Rep 2015;17(4):17.
105. Bonilla FA, Barlan I, Chapel H, et al. International consensus document (ICON): common variable immunodeficiency disorders. J Allergy Clin Immunol Pract 2016;4(1):38–59.
106. Bhan MK, Bhandari N, Bahl R. Management of the severely malnourished child: perspective from developing countries. BMJ 2003;326(7381):146–51.
107. Ochoa TJ, Salazar-Lindo E, Cleary TG. Management of children with infection-associated persistent diarrhea. Semin Pediatr Infect Dis 2004;15(4):229–36.
108. Di Costanzo M, Morelli M, Malamisura M, et al. Immunodeficiency disorders resulting in malabsorption. In: Guandalini S, Dhawan A, Branski D, editors. Textbook of pediatric gastroenterology, hepatology and nutrition: a comprehensive guide to practice. Cham (Switzerland): Springer International Publishing; 2016. p. 425–36.
109. Aslam A, Misbah SA, Talbot K, et al. Vitamin E deficiency induced neurological disease in common variable immunodeficiency: two cases and a review of the literature of vitamin E deficiency. Clin Immunol 2004;112(1):24–9.
110. Aukrust P, Müller F, Ueland T, et al. Decreased vitamin A levels in common variable immunodeficiency: vitamin A supplementation in vivo enhances immunoglobulin production and downregulates inflammatory responses. Eur J Clin Invest 2000;30(3):252–9.
111. Weizman Z, Binsztok M, Fraser D, et al. Intestinal protein loss in acute and persistent diarrhea of early childhood. J Clin Gastroenterol 2002;34(4):427–9.
112. Daniels JA, Torbenson M, Vivekanandan P, et al. Hepatitis in common variable immunodeficiency. Hum Pathol 2009;40(4):484–8.
113. Hernandez-Trujillo VP, Scalchunes C, Cunningham-Rundles C, et al. Autoimmunity and inflammation in X-linked agammaglobulinemia. J Clin Immunol 2014; 34(6):627–32.
114. Hanson EP, Monaco-Shawver L, Solt LA, et al. Hypomorphic nuclear factor-κB essential modulator mutation database and reconstitution system identifies phenotypic and immunologic diversity. J Allergy Clin Immunol 2008;122(6): 1169–77.e16.
115. Picard C, Casanova J-L, Puel A. Infectious diseases in patients with IRAK-4, MyD88, NEMO, or IκBα deficiency. Clin Microbiol Rev 2011;24(3):490–7.
116. Magnani A, Brosselin P, Beauté J, et al. Inflammatory manifestations in a single-center cohort of patients with chronic granulomatous disease. J Allergy Clin Immunol 2014;134(3):655–62.e8.
117. Alimchandani M, Lai J-P, Aung PP, et al. Gastrointestinal histopathology in chronic granulomatous disease – a study of 87 patients. Am J Surg Pathol 2013;37(9):1365–72.
118. Huang A, Abbasakoor F, Vaizey CJ. Gastrointestinal manifestations of chronic granulomatous disease. Colorectal Dis 2006;8(8):637–44.

119. Khangura SK, Kamal N, Ho N, et al. Gastrointestinal features of chronic granulomatous disease found during endoscopy. Clin Gastroenterol Hepatol 2016; 14(3):395–402.e5.
120. Moraes-Vasconcelos D, Costa-Carvalho BT, Torgerson TR, et al. Primary immune deficiency disorders presenting as autoimmune diseases: IPEX and APECED. J Clin Immunol 2008;28(Suppl 1):S11–9.
121. Rautemaa R, Hietanen J, Niissalo S, et al. Oral and oesophageal squamous cell carcinoma – a complication or component of autoimmune polyendocrinopathy-candidiasis-ectodermal dystrophy (APECED, APS-I). Oral Oncol 2007;43(6): 607–13.
122. Gambineri E, Perroni L, Passerini L, et al. Clinical and molecular profile of a new series of patients with immune dysregulation, polyendocrinopathy, enteropathy, X-linked syndrome: inconsistent correlation between forkhead box protein 3 expression and disease severity. J Allergy Clin Immunol 2008;122(6): 1105–12.e1.
123. Bennett CL, Christie J, Ramsdell F, et al. The immune dysregulation, polyendocrinopathy, enteropathy, X-linked syndrome (IPEX) is caused by mutations of FOXP3. Nat Genet 2001;27(1):20–1.
124. Barzaghi F, Passerini L, Bacchetta R. Immune dysregulation, polyendocrinopathy, enteropathy, x-linked syndrome: a paradigm of immunodeficiency with autoimmunity. Front Immunol 2012;3:211.
125. Verbsky JW, Chatila TA. Immune dysregulation, polyendocrinopathy, enteropathy, X-linked (IPEX) and IPEX-related disorders: an evolving web of heritable autoimmune diseases. Curr Opin Pediatr 2013;25(6):708–14.
126. Caudy AA, Reddy ST, Chatila T, et al. CD25 deficiency causes an immune dysregulation, polyendocrinopathy, enteropathy, X-linked–like syndrome, and defective IL-10 expression from CD4 lymphocytes. J Allergy Clin Immunol 2007;119(2):482–7.
127. Engelhardt KR, Shah N, Faizura-Yeop I, et al. Clinical outcome in IL-10– and IL-10 receptor–deficient patients with or without hematopoietic stem cell transplantation. J Allergy Clin Immunol 2013;131(3):825–30.
128. Kotlarz D, Beier R, Murugan D, et al. Loss of interleukin-10 signaling and infantile inflammatory bowel disease: implications for diagnosis and therapy. Gastroenterology 2012;143(2):347–55.
129. Yel L. Selective IgA deficiency. J Clin Immunol 2010;30(1):10–6.
130. Davies EG, Thrasher AJ. Update on the hyper immunoglobulin M syndromes. Br J Haematol 2010;149(2):167–80.
131. O'Gorman MRG, Zaas D, Paniagua M, et al. Development of a rapid whole blood flow cytometry procedure for the diagnosis of X-linked hyper-IgM syndrome patients and carriers. Clin Immunol Immunopathol 1997;85(2):172–81.
132. Lee W-I, Chen CC, Jaing TH, et al. A Nationwide study of severe and protracted diarrhoea in patients with primary immunodeficiency diseases. Sci Rep 2017; 7(1):3669.
133. Kobrynski LJ, Mayer L. Diagnosis and treatment of primary immunodeficiency disease in patients with gastrointestinal symptoms. Clin Immunol 2011;139(3): 238–48.
134. Marciano BE, Rosenzweig SD, Kleiner DE, et al. Gastrointestinal involvement in chronic granulomatous disease. Pediatrics 2004;114(2):462–8.
135. Marks DJB, Miyagi K, Rahman FZ, et al. Inflammatory bowel disease in CGD reproduces the clinicopathological features of Crohn's disease. Am J Gastroenterol 2008;104(1):117–24.

136. Yu JE, Azar AE, Chong HJ, et al. Considerations in the diagnosis of chronic granulomatous disease. J Pediatric Infect Dis Soc 2018;7(suppl_1):S6–11.

137. Rothblum-Oviatt C, Wright J, Lefton-Greif MA, et al. Ataxia telangiectasia: a review. Orphanet J Rare Dis 2016;11:159.

138. Staples ER, McDermott EM, Reiman A, et al. Immunodeficiency in ataxia telangiectasia is correlated strongly with the presence of two null mutations in the ataxia telangiectasia mutated gene. Clin Exp Immunol 2008;153(2):214–20.

139. Husebye ES, Perheentupa J, Rautemaa R, et al. Clinical manifestations and management of patients with autoimmune polyendocrine syndrome type I. J Intern Med 2009;265(5):514–29.

140. Chida N, Kobayashi I, Takezaki S, et al. Disease specificity of anti-tryptophan hydroxylase-1 and anti-AIE-75 autoantibodies in APECED and IPEX syndrome. Clin Immunol 2015;156(1):36–42.

141. Shah N, Kammermeier J, Elawad M, et al. Interleukin-10 and interleukin-10–receptor defects in inflammatory bowel disease. Curr Allergy Asthma Rep 2012; 12(5):373–9.

Gut Microbiome in Health and Disease
Emerging Diagnostic Opportunities

Aonghus Lavelle, MB, PhD[a], Colin Hill, MSc, PhD, DSc[b],*

KEYWORDS

- Microbiome • Colorectal cancer • Fecal microbiota transplantation
- Inflammatory bowel disease • Cancer immunotherapy • Personalized medicine
- Biomarkers

KEY POINTS

- Microbiome science has developed to the point where translation of pre-clinical observations into the clinical arena is imminent.
- Challenges facing the development of microbiome laboratory diagnostics include biological and environmental sources of variation, methodological standardization and the definition of health.
- Both gastrointestinal and extra-intestinal conditions are demonstrating great promise for microbiome-based diagnostics and therapeutics.
- Microbiome diagnostics may serve as biomarkers for disease risk or therapeutic efficacy, as companion diagnostics for microbiome-based therapies such as Fecal Microbiota Transplant or as a gateway to personalized interventions when integrated with other forms of personalized data.

INTRODUCTION

The gut microbiome encompasses the bacterial, viral, archaeal, fungal, and protozoal communities that live within our gastrointestinal tract. These communities significantly extend our complement of genes, allowing fermentation of otherwise inaccessible dietary food sources, providing a source of vitamins and allowing the metabolism of xenobiotics, in addition to playing a fundamental role in our metabolic homeostasis, immune education, and susceptibility to disease. However, numerous challenges have restricted our efforts to translate microbiome findings into routine diagnostic monitoring. Here, the authors describe the unique features of the microbiome that

Disclosure Statement: The authors have nothing to disclose.
[a] Department of Medicine, APC Microbiome Ireland, University College Cork, Cork, Ireland;
[b] School of Microbiology, APC Microbiome Ireland, University College Cork, Cork, Ireland
* Corresponding author.
E-mail address: c.hill@ucc.ie

Gastroenterol Clin N Am 48 (2019) 221–235
https://doi.org/10.1016/j.gtc.2019.02.003
0889-8553/19/© 2019 Elsevier Inc. All rights reserved.

make clinical translation a challenge and identify several key areas where early progress has been or is likely to be made.

ACQUISITION, ASSEMBLY, AND ESTABLISHED COMMUNITIES

At birth, humans rapidly become colonized with microbes in an essentially stochastic manner. Microbial exposure is essential for normal immune development, with a requirement for specific microbial functions at critical time points, the absence of which can lead to long-term effects on immune development.[1] Characteristic microbiomes based on body site are not present at birth,[2] with community structure and function rapidly consolidating to their respective niches by 6 weeks of age.[3] Although most neonatal body sites and fluids resemble maternal skin and vaginal communities, meconium, the first pass of intestinal contents, has a distinct microbial composition, which may suggest that limited first microbial contact may actually occur in utero.[4]

Succession of gut microbial species toward an adult microbiome takes place over the following 1 to 3 years[5] and is almost certainly influenced by preterm delivery and antibiotic use,[6] feeding,[7] maternal health,[8] and delivery mode.[9] Succession of bacterial communities is a nonrandom process, with changes in diet, particularly discontinuation of breast feeding[5] and the commencement of solid foods resulting in defined transitions, an increase in diversity, and convergence toward an adult configuration.[10]

By adulthood, the distal gut microbiome contains an estimated 10^{10} to 10^{11} bacteria per gram of feces,[11] dominated by the phyla Bacteroidetes and Firmicutes, with varying contributions from other phyla, including Proteobacteria, Actinobacteria, and Verrucomicrobia.[12] Combined data from the Flemish Gut Flora Project, the LLDeep cohort in Holland, the human microbiome project (HMP), and the UK twins study described 664 genera, with an estimate of 784 $\pm$ 40 genera total richness in western populations.[13] Adding data from New Guinea, Peru, and Tanzania, 14 core genera were present in greater than 95% of individuals across the dataset, suggesting a global core bacterial microbiome.

NONBACTERIAL COMPONENTS

In addition to bacteria, large communities of viruses exist within the gut microbiome. Bacteriophages, viruses with a bacterial host, dominate this population and exist at approximately 10^{10} to 10^{11} particles per gram of feces,[14] with potentially higher quantities on mucosal surfaces.[15] In ecological communities, such as marine environments, phage and their hosts interact in a cycle of bacterial infection, replication, cell lysis, and resistance, leading to an evolutionary "arms race." This lytic cycle contrasts with the predominant behavior of phages within the gut, where a temperate or lysogenic cycle leads to incorporation of phage DNA within the host genome, reverting to lytic behavior under certain stresses.[16] Phages can thus have direct and indirect effects on their host communities.[17] Succession dynamics,[18] temporal stability,[19] and interindividual variation[20] appear broadly similar to bacterial communities, and although the complete role of phages within the gut remains to be determined, they have been associated with certain disease, including inflammatory bowel disease (IBD),[21] and show potential as biomarkers and therapeutic tools.[22]

Microbial eukaryotes, such as diverse fungal species, are also important and are biologically relevant, although accounting for a numerically small portion of the total microbial community. The gut "mycobiome" is dominated by yeast, prominently Saccharomyces, Malassezia, and Candida spp in the HMP cohort, and overall, fungal communities are less diverse.[23] Decreases in certain fungal species with anti-inflammatory properties, such as Saccharomyces cerevisiae, as well as increases in potentially pathogenic species, such as *Candida albicans*, have been described in IBD.[24] Interestingly, less temporal stability is observed in terms of fungal communities with a loss of significant interpersonal differentiation over time, contrasting with the case of the gut bacteriome and virome.[23]

SOURCES OF MICROBIOME VARIATION
Biological and Environmental

In terms of the human-associated microbiome, the largest variation in taxonomic composition is consistently between body habitats, whereas within body habitats, there is a large degree of interpersonal variation, as evidenced by the findings of the Human Microbiome Project,[12] with individuals also tending to remain more like themselves than others over time.[25] However, when viewed in terms of the genetic composition of the microbiome, this striking interindividual variation largely disappears, highlighting that the underlying genetic machinery is much more tightly conserved.

Interpersonal variability does not appear to be strongly shaped by host genetic makeup or microbiome heritability but is markedly influenced by environmental exposures, as recently demonstrated in a large Israeli cohort and validated in a Dutch population.[26] In this landmark study, microbiome composition was additive with host genotype in predicting a range of host phenotypes, including blood markers of glycemic control and high-density lipoprotein cholesterol, body mass index (BMI), and several anthropometric measures. Factors that have been demonstrated to have an association with microbiome composition include diet, stool consistency, medication use, antibiotic prescribing, BMI, household sharing, blood parameters, gender, health, physical activity, and age; these are essential covariates for any large microbiome study[13,26,27] (**Fig. 1A**).

Methodological

In addition to biological variation, variation in technical approach is a significant obstacle to comparability between studies (**Fig. 1B**). Various DNA sequencing methodologies have been used, including 454 pyrosequencing and Illumina technologies, whereas third-generation sequencing platforms are emerging, such as PacBio and MinION.[28] At the other end of the spectrum, polymerase chain reaction (PCR) can identify specific members of the community, whereas in between, microarray technology has been used to develop the HITchip, a fixed phylogenetic array.[29] In addition, agreed protocols for acquisition, storage, DNA extraction, amplification, sequencing, and bioinformatic analysis of biological samples are beginning to be published. To tackle variations between approaches, the Microbiome Quality Control Project (www.mbqc.org/) has published their first round of protocols for the handling and bioinformatic analysis of metagenomic and amplicon sequencing of gut samples.[30,31] Notably, DNA extraction, handling laboratory and bioinformatics pipeline all have effects, at times comparable to biological sources of variation. Bioinformatic approaches have also been applied to the important issue of microbial contamination, and a Bayesian method, SourceTracker, has been developed.[32] It should be noted that variation in methodologies is to be expected in a rapidly developing area, and it is important that standardization does not impede innovations in method development.

DEFINING HEALTH

One of the major challenges in microbiome science (and other areas of medicine) involves defining health. Given the sources of variation described above and the

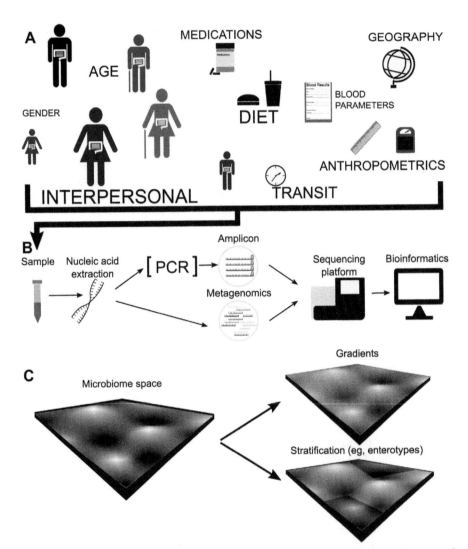

Fig. 1. (A) Biological and environmental sources of variation. (B) Methodological sources of variation. (C) Representation of the microbiome landscape, with alternate interpretations of gradients or stratification (equivalent to enterotypes).

"landscape of possible microbiome configurations,"[33] this has been challenging (**Fig. 1C**). Enterotypes, defined as "densely populated areas in a multidimensional space of community composition," were associated initially with 1 of 3 key indicator taxons, namely *Prevotella*, *Bacteroides*, or *Ruminococcaceae*.[34] Definition of these densely populated areas does depend on the statistical methodology applied and may change with geographic source, reflecting data biased in favor of Western countries.[33,34] However, enterotypes, particularly those associated with *Prevotella* and *Bacteroides*, have been widely reproduced, demonstrate enterotype-specific enrichments of functional gene categories, and have been associated with host disease phenotypes.[33] Such a proposal allows for stratification of individuals and may facilitate numerous clinical applications, including biomarker discovery and personalized interventions. However, further large-scale studies are required to determine if different enterotypes are linked to meaningful clinical differences. In addition, as de novo clustering is dependent on the current sample set, potential clinical applications require a reference "enterotype-space" to assure samples are correctly assigned to their true cluster. In discovery projects, ordination results are highly dependent on the statistical method applied, the number of samples, and the sequence coverage,[35] and underlying all these efforts remains the requirement for strict standardization of sample acquisition and processing in studies that are to be directly compared with one another.

Although enterotypes provide a mechanism of recovering structure across the microbiome landscape, direct comparison between disease and health in case-control studies remains an important tool for identifying disease-associated microbiome alterations. Many disease-associated confounders exist however, as demonstrated in the case of type II diabetes mellitus (T2DM), where the purported disease-associated alterations were subsequently attributed to metformin, a common oral hypoglycemic agent used in the treatment of T2DM.[36] A large Flemish population study (the Flemish Gut Flora Project) has estimated that between 400 and 900 individuals per group would be required to adequately power microbiome studies depending on the circumstance and background covariates.[13] These results suggest that many studies comparing disease and control subjects are underpowered, leading to the conclusions that reference datasets with heavily phenotyped control subjects for matching will be invaluable for future microbiome discovery projects.

CLINICAL OPPORTUNITIES

Although the factors detailed above represent significant challenges to universal diagnostic microbiome tests, certain clinical scenarios show great promise for translational applications. The authors describe several of these, in both gastrointestinal and non-gastrointestinal disorders, to illustrate the scope and application of potential microbiome-based diagnostics (**Box 1**).

Colorectal Cancer

Although clinically isolated strains of gut bacteria, such as *Streptococcus bovis* bacteremia, have been associated with colorectal cancer (CRC),[37] culture-independent sequencing technologies have provided many insights into compositional changes

---

Box 1
Opportunities for microbiome-based diagnostics

Microbiome-based biomarkers may improve population screening for colorectal cancer and precancerous lesions.

Microbiome-based diagnostics may inform therapeutic pathways in CD, particularly suitability for treatment deescalation and risk-stratification for postoperative recurrence.

Coupling microbiome diagnostics and therapeutics will become important, particularly in the era of FMT and may aid rational matching of donors-recipients in clinical trials for IBD.

Identification of patients with cancer at risk of nonresponse to immunotherapy and subsequent expansion of specific bacterial populations may improve response rates to checkpoint inhibitors.

Personalized dietary interventions, incorporating microbiome analysis, represent a prototype for integrated approaches to personalized therapeutics.

associated with CRC, and there is mounting evidence to suggest that the intestinal microbiota may play a key role in its pathogenesis. Specific bacteria that have been associated with CRC tumorigenesis include *Escherichia coli*,[38] enterotoxigenic *Bacteroides fragilis*,[39] and, most commonly, *Fusobacterium nucleatum*.

F nucleatum is an invasive gram-negative bacterium, important in polymicrobial biofilms associated with periodontitis,[40] and is notably also increased in IBD, where it may be more invasive.[41] *F nucleatum* has been found to be increased in CRC,[42,43] precancerous lesions,[44,45] and fecal samples in CRC[46] and has even been detected in CRC metastases.[43] *Fusobacterium* carriage may also have prognostic relevance and has been associated with lymph-node metastases[42,47] and reduced overall survival.[48,49] These findings have strong mechanistic underpinnings, with *F nucleatum* known to activate β-catenin signaling via a surface adhesin, FadA, binding to E-cadherin. Furthermore, *F nucleatum* can enhance progression of tumors by causing an increase in tumor-infiltrating myeloid cells within the tumor microenvironment.[50,51] Despite this, it is likely that *Fusobacterium* spp are only associated with a subset of CRCs.[43]

Other associations with oral pathogens have also been demonstrated. Using a Dirichlet Multinomial Model, investigators in China identified 5 metacommunities associated with different phenotypes (controls, adenomas, and CRC). Interestingly, the metacommunity with the strongest association with CRC was characterized by enrichment of *F nucleatum* and other periodontal pathogens.[52] Associations with periodontal disease and CRC have been described,[53] and increased prevalence of pathogenic oral bacteria groups, including *Peptostreptococcus*, *Prevotella*, *Steptococcus*, *Parvimonas*, and *Porphyromonas*, has been associated with reduced colonic abundance of *Lachnospiraceae*.[54,55]

These findings allowed investigators to demonstrate that microbiome-based screening can supplement current noninvasive biomarkers, such as fecal occult blood (FOB)[56] tests or fecal immunohistochemical tests (FIT),[54] to improve detection of early colorectal neoplasia (**Fig. 2A**). Using quantitative PCR of the butyryl-CoA dehydrogenase gene from *F nucleatum* and the rpoB gene from *Parvimonas micra* determined by cross-ethnic validation, investigators achieved a true-positive detection rate (TPR) of 0.723 with a false-positive rate (FPR) of 0.073 without the use of FOB or FIT.[57] Adding oral microbiota to stool allowed Irish researchers to improve detection of CRC, with a TPR of 0.76 and an FPR of 0.05.[55]

Therapeutic Strategies in Crohn's Disease

Many studies have demonstrated microbiome alterations associated with IBD, most prominently Crohn's disease (CD), and specifically, ileal CD, with a common theme being a reduction in overall bacterial diversity.[58] Reductions in butyrate-producing species, particularly *Faecalibacterium prausnitzii* in CD[58,59] as well as selected members of the *Lachnospiraceae*,[58] have been consistently described, with increases in adherent and invasive *E coli* demonstrated in the ileum of ileal CD patients.[60] Increased prevalence of *Ruminococcus gnavus*, Proteobacteria, *Veillonella*, and *Fusobacterium* spp has also been described.[61,62] Notably, children with new onset CD before treatment demonstrated much more dramatic microbiome alterations when mucosal biopsy samples were sequenced compared with stool samples, with predictive power for 6-month disease activity, suggesting that the diagnostic and prognostic viability of microbiome-based biomarkers in IBD may be enhanced by mucosal biopsy sampling.[62]

Microbiome analysis has also demonstrated efficacy in predicting anastomotic recurrence of CD following surgical resection,[63] a common problem that can affect

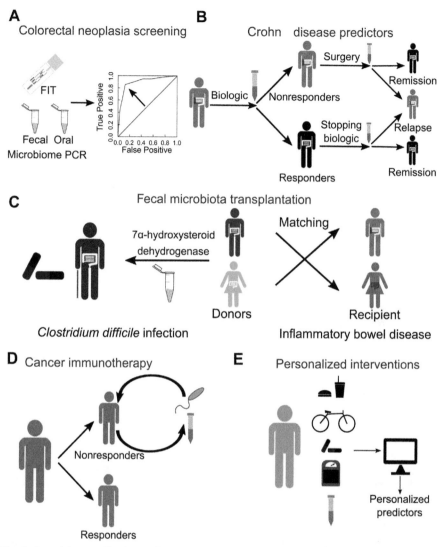

Fig. 2. Promising applications of microbiome-based diagnostics based on seminal research findings discussed in the text. (*A*) Improving sensitivity and specificity of noninvasive colorectal neoplasia detection. (*B*) Potential microbiome predictors in CD. (*C*) Applications of FMT in CDI and IBD. (*D*) Microbiome assessment as a potential source of nonresponse in cancer immunotherapy with potential for targeted modulation. (*E*) Integrating personalized microbiome data with other data types to develop personalized prediction algorithms.

more than half of patients who undergo this procedure and occurs following restoration of the fecal stream[64] (**Fig. 2B**). Recovery of mucosal microbiome composition at 6-months postsurgery was associated with remission, while putative fecal biomarkers of disease recurrence presurgery were also noted.[63] In addition, in a parallel evaluation of the pivotal POCER (Post-Operative Crohn's Disease Recurrence) study, evaluating strategies for preventing postoperative recurrence of CD, levels of *Faecalibacterium* and *Proteus*, in combination with smoking status, were moderately predictive of early recurrence.[65]

In a therapeutic setting, PCR-based microbiome analysis predicted relapse independently of the inflammatory marker CRP following withdrawal of therapy with infliximab in CD, a question of huge clinical relevance given the cost and potential side effects of long-term biologic therapy.[66] More recently, in a multiethnic Chinese and Western cohort, microbial species could predict response to infliximab therapy with 86.5% accuracy, improving to 93.8% when combined with the stool marker fecal calprotectin.[67] These findings are extremely promising in identifying microbiome-based diagnostics, which are additive with markers of inflammatory burden that have traditionally been associated with response prediction.

Fecal Microbiota Transplantation

Fecal microbiota transplantation (FMT) has become a standard treatment of recurrent *Clostridium difficile* infection (CDI), a major health care challenge associated with antibiotic use.[68] Recurrent CDI occurs in approximately 20% of CDI cases, associated with a marked loss of microbiome diversity and an inability of the native microbiome to "reboot" following treatment of CDI with specific antibiotics, such as vancomycin, metronidazole, and fidaxomicin. Just a single dose of the antibiotic clindamycin results in a profound loss of diversity in the gut microbiota of mice and a resulting enhanced susceptibility to CDI,[69] presumably because of the commensal microbiota providing a significant barrier via colonization resistance. First-line antibiotic treatments, such as vancomycin, can result in profound and persistent collateral effects on the microbiome, which may be associated with subsequent risk of pathogen expansion and is remediated by FMT.[70] FMT is commonly performed at endoscopy, where healthy donor fecal suspensions that have been prescreened for pathogens are infused into the recipient. Donor feces can be acquired from healthy volunteers or increasingly from donor banks, such as OpenBiome. Extensive screening of donor samples is required to prevent pathogen transmission, and extended host phenotype exclusion criteria and standardized screening protocols will become important.[71] Phase 3 clinical trials on commercially prepared products are also underway, including SER-109, a capsule made by Seres Therapeutics, and RBX2660, an enema bag made by Rebiotix.

Incorporating microbiome parameters into models has also helped improve classification of CDI, and a combination of clinical and microbiome variables may better predict at-risk hospitalized patients.[72] Furthermore, specific molecular mechanisms have been elucidated, identifying that the microbiota also provides resistance to CDI through bile acid metabolism.[73] Investigators have identified loss of a specific bacterial species, *Clostridium scindens*, which provides colonization resistance to CDI due to expression of the secondary bile acid biosynthesis gene, 7α-hydroxysteroid dehydrogenase, detectable by PCR.[74] Recovery of resistance to CDI occurred with administration of this bacterium, pointing toward a potential combination of PCR-based diagnosis and targeted therapeutic expansion (**Fig. 2C**).

FMT is also being investigated in other conditions, notably IBD. Some promise has been demonstrated in ulcerative colitis, where several randomized controlled trials have demonstrated variable efficacy in induction of remission,[75–77] although not all.[78] Interestingly, the potential for certain healthy donors to be better at inducing remission was suggested ("superdonors"). Higher donor richness,[79] the presence of conspecific or shared species,[80] and increased butyrate production, with lower levels of Bacteroidetes and Proteobacteria in donors,[81] were associated with induction of remission, suggesting that refined selection of donors and potential matching strategies may improve remission rates.

Cancer Immunotherapy

The gut microbiome plays a fundamental role in the education of innate and adaptive immune responses as well as in maintenance of immune homeostasis. Cancer immunotherapy seeks to inhibit tumor-derived immunosuppression via immune checkpoint inhibitors against programmed cell death protein-1 (PD-1) and its ligand, PD-L1, as well as CTLA-4, although response rates are variable. In patients treated with checkpoint inhibitors, response phenotype can be transferred to germ-free mice from patients by fecal transplant, suggesting a pivotal role for the microbiome in clinical response to immunotherapy.[82] Germ-free or antibiotic-treated murine cancer models show a significantly reduced response to a range of chemotherapeutic and anticancer treatments, whereas in humans, a reduction in the efficacy of PD-1/PD-L1 inhibitors has been demonstrated following antibiotic administration across a range of cancer types. Specific bacteria associated with response include the presence of *Akkermansia muciniphila*, *Alistipes*, and members of the Firmicutes.[83] Similar findings have been reported for CTLA-4 inhibitors, although this was associated with specific *Bacteroides* species, notably *B fragilis*.[84] Further associations include increased presence of *Enterococcus hirae* in response to both PD-1/PD-L1 inhibition and cyclophosphamide therapy.[85] In another seminal study, melanoma xenograft mice (C57Bl/6) demonstrated differences in tumor growth rate depending on vendor, attributable to differences in intratumoral T-cell response.[86] Cohousing, or appropriately directed transplant of fecal suspensions, could ameliorate the effects on tumor growth and tumor immune response. *Bifidobacterium* was most strongly associated with an increased immune response; therapeutic administration of *Bifidobacterium* species from different sources reduced tumor growth. *Bifidobacterium longum* was also found to be increased in responders to checkpoint inhibitors, in addition to *Collinsella aerofaciens* and *Enterococcus faecium*.[82] Although there is a lack of consistency between studies as to which bacterial species mediate these effects, multiple lines of evidence point toward microbiome-mediated response to immunotherapy in cancer, opening the door to a promising field of coupled diagnostic and therapeutic interventions to improve response to cancer immunotherapy[87] (**Fig. 2D**).

Personalized Dietary Interventions

Host metabolism is intrinsically linked to the gut microbiome, and numerous foundational studies have demonstrated that the microbiome plays a key role in energy harvest, obesity, and metabolic syndrome.[88–90] As described throughout this review, interpersonal variation is consistently the most significant variable in terms of gut microbiome composition. Researchers in Israel have demonstrated that postprandial glycemic response (PPGR) is also highly variable between individuals.[91] Using a cohort of more than 800 individuals with continuous blood glucose tracking, combined with dietary, lifestyle, medical, anthropometric, and microbiome analysis, the researchers were able to predict PPGR using a machine-learning algorithm far more accurately than by meal carbohydrate content. The improved prediction of PPGR was validated in a subsequent cohort and was the basis of a successful trial, where personalized diets were comparable when administered by an expert or by the algorithm. Both the expert and the algorithm had access to continuous glucose monitoring data for the prior week, although only the algorithm could make inferences about previously unobserved meals, while additionally being able to leverage information on other lifestyle covariates. Interestingly, despite the variation in microbiome composition between individuals, some conserved patterns were noted in response to the short-term dietary intervention (which involved 1 week of a "good" diet and 1 week of a "bad" diet), including increases in *Roseburia inulinivorans*, *Eubacterium eligens*, *Alistipes putredinis*, and *Bacteroides vulgatus* and reductions in *Bifidobacterium adolescentis* and Anaerostipes following the "good" diet, largely consistent with previous literature. In a smaller study looking at white bread in comparison to sourdough bread, the same group demonstrated similar findings, although in this case, they were able to accurately predict PPGR based on initial microbiome composition alone.[92]

These pivotal studies have demonstrated that interpersonal variation in the microbiome can be a gateway into personalized dietary interventions, with an enormous potential for extension into personalized diagnostics and therapeutics (**Fig. 2E**). Importantly, they also provide a template for the manner in which data from microbiome studies may be integrated with lifestyle, dietary, and medical data, to provide a personalized model of microbiome and host response to interventions.

SUMMARY

A new horizon of microbiome-based diagnostic tools is in sight, ranging from assays to improve noninvasive population screening in conditions like CRC, to complementary biomarkers of disease progression and therapeutic response in IBD. Focused microbiome analysis may help identify individuals at risk of CDI and allow for targeted rescue of colonization resistance, as well as informing rational matching strategies for emerging FMT indications, such as in IBD. More broadly, extensive microbiome characterization may be integrated into a personalized portfolio of features, allowing for tailored intervention strategies in a range of conditions. Large-scale population cohorts, adequately powered studies, applications of data science, and universal standardization of pipelines will be required to realize these ambitious goals in the coming years.

ACKNOWLEDGEMENTS

APC Microbiome Ireland is funded with financial support by Science Foundation Ireland (SFI) under Grant Number SFI/12/RC/2273.

REFERENCES

1. Gomez de Aguero M, Ganal-Vonarburg SC, Fuhrer T, et al. The maternal microbiota drives early postnatal innate immune development. Science 2016; 351(6279):1296–302.
2. Dominguez-Bello MG, Costello EK, Contreras M, et al. Delivery mode shapes the acquisition and structure of the initial microbiota across multiple body habitats in newborns. Proc Natl Acad Sci U S A 2010;107(26):11971–5.
3. Chu DM, Ma J, Prince AL, et al. Maturation of the infant microbiome community structure and function across multiple body sites and in relation to mode of delivery. Nat Med 2017;23:314.
4. Collado MC, Rautava S, Aakko J, et al. Human gut colonisation may be initiated in utero by distinct microbial communities in the placenta and amniotic fluid. Sci Rep 2016;6:23129.
5. Bäckhed F, Roswall J, Peng Y, et al. Dynamics and stabilization of the human gut microbiome during the first year of life. Cell Host Microbe 2015;17(6):852.
6. Gibson MK, Wang B, Ahmadi S, et al. Developmental dynamics of the preterm infant gut microbiota and antibiotic resistome. Nat Microbiol 2016;1:16024.
7. Bokulich NA, Chung J, Battaglia T, et al. Antibiotics, birth mode, and diet shape microbiome maturation during early life. Sci Transl Med 2016;8(343):343ra82.

8. Hu J, Nomura Y, Bashir A, et al. Diversified microbiota of meconium is affected by maternal diabetes status. PLoS One 2013;8(11):e78257.

9. Azad MB, Konya T, Maughan H, et al. Gut microbiota of healthy Canadian infants: profiles by mode of delivery and infant diet at 4 months. CMAJ 2013;185(5): 385–94.

10. Koenig JE, Spor A, Scalfone N, et al. Succession of microbial consortia in the developing infant gut microbiome. Proc Natl Acad Sci U S A 2011;108(Suppl 1):4578–85.

11. Vandeputte D, Kathagen G, D'Hoe K, et al. Quantitative microbiome profiling links gut community variation to microbial load. Nature 2017;551(7681):507–11.

12. The Human Microbiome Consortium. Structure, function and diversity of the healthy human microbiome. Nature 2012;486(7402):207–14.

13. Falony G, Joossens M, Vieira-Silva S, et al. Population-level analysis of gut microbiome variation. Science 2016;352(6285):560–4.

14. Shkoporov AN, Ryan FJ, Draper LA, et al. Reproducible protocols for metagenomic analysis of human faecal phageomes. Microbiome 2018;6(1):68.

15. Barr JJ, Auro R, Furlan M, et al. Bacteriophage adhering to mucus provide a non-host-derived immunity. Proc Natl Acad Sci U S A 2013;110(26):10771–6.

16. Fuhrman JA. Marine viruses and their biogeochemical and ecological effects. Nature 1999;399:541.

17. Manrique P, Dills M, Young M. The human gut phage community and its implications for health and disease. Viruses 2017;9(6):141.

18. Breitbart M, Haynes M, Kelley S, et al. Viral diversity and dynamics in an infant gut. Res Microbiol 2008;159(5):367–73.

19. Minot S, Bryson A, Chehoud C, et al. Rapid evolution of the human gut virome. Proc Natl Acad Sci U S A 2013;110(30):12450–5.

20. Minot S, Sinha R, Chen J, et al. The human gut virome: inter-individual variation and dynamic response to diet. Genome Res 2011;21(10):1616–25.

21. Norman JM, Handley SA, Baldridge MT, et al. Disease-specific alterations in the enteric virome in inflammatory bowel disease. Cell 2015;160(3):447–60.

22. Dalmasso M, Hill C, Ross RP. Exploiting gut bacteriophages for human health. Trends Microbiol 2014;22(7):399–405.

23. Nash AK, Auchtung TA, Wong MC, et al. The gut mycobiome of the Human Microbiome Project healthy cohort. Microbiome 2017;5:153.

24. Sokol H, Leducq V, Aschard H, et al. Fungal microbiota dysbiosis in IBD. Gut 2017;66(6):1039–48.

25. Costello EK, Lauber CL, Hamady M, et al. Bacterial community variation in human body habitats across space and time. Science 2009;326(5960):1694–7.

26. Rothschild D, Weissbrod O, Barkan E, et al. Environment dominates over host genetics in shaping human gut microbiota. Nature 2018;555:210.

27. Maier L, Pruteanu M, Kuhn M, et al. Extensive impact of non-antibiotic drugs on human gut bacteria. Nature 2018;555:623.

28. Cao Y, Fanning S, Proos S, et al. A review on the applications of next generation sequencing technologies as applied to food-related microbiome studies. Front Microbiol 2017;8:1829.

29. Rajilić-Stojanović M, Heilig HGHJ, Molenaar D, et al. Development and application of the human intestinal tract chip, a phylogenetic microarray: analysis of universally conserved phylotypes in the abundant microbiota of young and elderly adults. Environ Microbiol 2009;11(7):1736–51.

30. Sinha R, Abu-Ali G, Vogtmann E, et al. Assessment of variation in microbial community amplicon sequencing by the Microbiome Quality Control (MBQC) project consortium. Nat Biotechnol 2017;35(11):1077–86.

31. Costea PI, Zeller G, Sunagawa S, et al. Towards standards for human fecal sample processing in metagenomic studies. Nat Biotechnol 2017;35(11):1069–76.

32. Knights D, Kuczynski J, Charlson ES, et al. Bayesian community-wide culture-independent microbial source tracking. Nat Methods 2011;8(9):761–3.

33. Costea PI, Hildebrand F, Arumugam M, et al. Enterotypes in the landscape of gut microbial community composition. Nat Microbiol 2018;3(1):8–16.

34. Arumugam M, Raes J, Pelletier E, et al. Enterotypes of the human gut microbiome. Nature 2011;473(7346):174–80.

35. Kuczynski J, Liu Z, Lozupone C, et al. Microbial community resemblance methods differ in their ability to detect biologically relevant patterns. Nat Methods 2010;7(10):813–9.

36. Forslund K, Hildebrand F, Nielsen T, et al. Disentangling type 2 diabetes and metformin treatment signatures in the human gut microbiota. Nature 2015;528:262.

37. Corredoira JC, Alonso MP, Garcia JF, et al. Clinical characteristics and significance of Streptococcus salivarius bacteremia and Streptococcus bovis bacteremia: a prospective 16-year study. Eur J Clin Microbiol Infect Dis 2005;24(4): 250–5.

38. Arthur JC, Perez-Chanona E, Mühlbauer M, et al. Intestinal inflammation targets cancer-inducing activity of the microbiota. Science 2012;338(6103):120–3.

39. Toprak NU, Yagci A, Gulluoglu BM, et al. A possible role of Bacteroides fragilis enterotoxin in the aetiology of colorectal cancer. Clin Microbiol Infect 2006; 12(8):782–6.

40. Signat B, Roques C, Poulet P, et al. Fusobacterium nucleatum in periodontal health and disease. Curr Issues Mol Biol 2011;13(2):25–36.

41. Strauss J, Kaplan GG, Beck PL, et al. Invasive potential of gut mucosa-derived Fusobacterium nucleatum positively correlates with IBD status of the host. Inflamm Bowel Dis 2011;17(9):1971–8.

42. Castellarin M, Warren RL, Freeman JD, et al. Fusobacterium nucleatum infection is prevalent in human colorectal carcinoma. Genome Res 2012;22(2):299–306.

43. Kostic AD, Gevers D, Pedamallu CS, et al. Genomic analysis identifies association of Fusobacterium with colorectal carcinoma. Genome Res 2012;22(2):292–8.

44. McCoy AN, Araújo-Pérez F, Azcárate-Peril A, et al. Fusobacterium is associated with colorectal adenomas. PLoS One 2013;8(1):e53653.

45. Miki I, Shinichi K, Katsuhiko N, et al. Association of Fusobacterium nucleatum with clinical and molecular features in colorectal serrated pathway. Int J Cancer 2015; 137(6):1258–68.

46. Ahn J, Sinha R, Pei Z, et al. Human gut microbiome and risk for colorectal cancer. J Natl Cancer Inst 2013;105(24):1907–11.

47. Li YY, Ge QX, Cao J, et al. Association of Fusobacterium nucleatum infection with colorectal cancer in Chinese patients. World J Gastroenterol 2016;22(11): 3227–33.

48. Flanagan L, Schmid J, Ebert M, et al. Fusobacterium nucleatum associates with stages of colorectal neoplasia development, colorectal cancer and disease outcome. Eur J Clin Microbiol Infect Dis 2014;33(8):1381–90.

49. Mima K, Nishihara R, Qian ZR, et al. Fusobacterium nucleatum in colorectal carcinoma tissue and patient prognosis. Gut 2016;65(12):1973–80.

50. Rubinstein Mara R, Wang X, Liu W, et al. *Fusobacterium nucleatum* promotes colorectal carcinogenesis by modulating E-Cadherin/β-Catenin signaling via its FadA adhesin. Cell Host Microbe 2013;14(2):195–206.

51. Kostic Aleksandar D, Chun E, Robertson L, et al. *Fusobacterium nucleatum* potentiates intestinal tumorigenesis and modulates the tumor-immune microenvironment. Cell Host Microbe 2013;14(2):207–15.

52. Nakatsu G, Li X, Zhou H, et al. Gut mucosal microbiome across stages of colorectal carcinogenesis. Nat Commun 2015;6:8727.

53. Momen-Heravi F, Babic A, Tworoger SS, et al. Periodontal disease, tooth loss and colorectal cancer risk: results from the Nurses' Health Study. Int J Cancer 2017; 140(3):646–52.

54. Baxter NT, Ruffin MT, Rogers MA, et al. Microbiota-based model improves the sensitivity of fecal immunochemical test for detecting colonic lesions. Genome Med 2016;8(1):37.

55. Flemer B, Warren RD, Barrett MP, et al. The oral microbiota in colorectal cancer is distinctive and predictive. Gut 2018;67(8):1454–63.

56. Zeller G, Tap J, Voigt AY, et al. Potential of fecal microbiota for early-stage detection of colorectal cancer. Mol Syst Biol 2014;10(11):766.

57. Yu J, Feng Q, Wong SH, et al. Metagenomic analysis of faecal microbiome as a tool towards targeted non-invasive biomarkers for colorectal cancer. Gut 2017; 66(1):70–8.

58. Willing BP, Dicksved J, Halfvarson J, et al. A pyrosequencing study in twins shows that gastrointestinal microbial profiles vary with inflammatory bowel disease phenotypes. Gastroenterology 2010;139(6):1844–54.e1.

59. Sokol H, Pigneur B, Watterlot L, et al. Faecalibacterium prausnitzii is an anti-inflammatory commensal bacterium identified by gut microbiota analysis of Crohn's disease patients. Proc Natl Acad Sci U S A 2008;105(43):16731–6.

60. Darfeuille-Michaud A, Boudeau J, Bulois P, et al. High prevalence of adherent-invasive Escherichia coli associated with ileal mucosa in Crohn's disease. Gastroenterology 2004;127(2):412–21.

61. Quince C, Ijaz UZ, Loman N, et al. Extensive modulation of the fecal metagenome in children with Crohn's disease during exclusive enteral nutrition. Am J Gastroenterol 2015;110(12):1718–29 [quiz: 1730].

62. Gevers D, Kugathasan S, Denson LA, et al. The treatment-naive microbiome in new-onset Crohn's disease. Cell Host Microbe 2014;15(3):382–92.

63. Mondot S, Lepage P, Seksik P, et al. Structural robustness of the gut mucosal microbiota is associated with Crohn's disease remission after surgery. Gut 2016; 65(6):954–62.

64. D'Haens GR, Geboes K, Peeters M, et al. Early lesions of recurrent Crohn's disease caused by infusion of intestinal contents in excluded ileum. Gastroenterology 1998;114(2):262–7.

65. Wright EK, Kamm MA, Wagner J, et al. Microbial factors associated with postoperative Crohn's disease recurrence. J Crohn's Colitis 2017;11(2):191–203.

66. Rajca S, Grondin V, Louis E, et al. Alterations in the intestinal microbiome (dysbiosis) as a predictor of relapse after infliximab withdrawal in Crohn's disease. Inflamm Bowel Dis 2014;20(6):978–86.

67. Zhou Y, Xu ZZ, He Y, et al. Gut microbiota offers universal biomarkers across ethnicity in inflammatory bowel disease diagnosis and infliximab response prediction. mSystems 2018;3(1) [pii:e00188-17].

68. van Nood E, Vrieze A, Nieuwdorp M, et al. Duodenal infusion of donor feces for recurrent Clostridium difficile. N Engl J Med 2013;368(5):407–15.

69. Buffie CG, Jarchum I, Equinda M, et al. Profound alterations of intestinal micro-biota following a single dose of clindamycin results in sustained susceptibility to Clostridium difficile-induced colitis. Infect Immun 2012;80(1):62–73.
70. Isaac S, Scher JU, Djukovic A, et al. Short- and long-term effects of oral vanco-mycin on the human intestinal microbiota. J Antimicrob Chemother 2017;72(1): 128–36.
71. Ding NS, Mullish BH, McLaughlin J, et al. Meeting update: faecal microbiota transplantation—bench, bedside, courtroom? Frontline Gastroenterol 2018;9(1): 45–8.
72. Schubert AM, Rogers MAM, Ring C, et al. Microbiome data distinguish patients with Clostridium difficile infection and Non-C. difficile-associated diarrhea from healthy controls. MBio 2014;5(3). e01021-14.
73. Weingarden AR, Chen C, Bobr A, et al. Microbiota transplantation restores normal fecal bile acid composition in recurrent Clostridium difficile infection. Am J Physiol Gastrointest Liver Physiol 2014;306(4):G310–9.
74. Buffie CG, Bucci V, Stein RR, et al. Precision microbiome reconstitution restores bile acid mediated resistance to Clostridium difficile. Nature 2015;517(7533): 205–8.
75. Moayyedi P, Surette MG, Kim PT, et al. Fecal microbiota transplantation induces remission in patients with active ulcerative colitis in a randomized controlled trial. Gastroenterology 2015;149(1):102–9.e6.
76. Paramsothy S, Kamm MA, Kaakoush NO, et al. Multidonor intensive faecal micro-biota transplantation for active ulcerative colitis: a randomised placebo-controlled trial. Lancet 2017;389(10075):1218–28.
77. Costello SP, Waters O, Bryant RV, et al. Short duration, low intensity, pooled fecal microbiota transplantation induces remission in patients with mild-moderately active ulcerative colitis: a randomised controlled trial. Gastroenterology 2017; 152(5):S198–9.
78. Rossen NG, Fuentes S, van der Spek MJ, et al. Findings from a randomized controlled trial of fecal transplantation for patients with ulcerative colitis. Gastro-enterology 2015;149(1):110–8.e4.
79. Vermeire S, Joossens M, Verbeke K, et al. Donor species richness determines faecal microbiota transplantation success in inflammatory bowel disease. J Crohn's Colitis 2016;10(4):387–94.
80. Li SS, Zhu A, Benes V, et al. Durable coexistence of donor and recipient strains after fecal microbiota transplantation. Science 2016;352(6285):586–9.
81. Fuentes S, Rossen NG, van der Spek MJ, et al. Microbial shifts and signatures of long-term remission in ulcerative colitis after faecal microbiota transplantation. ISME J 2017;11(8):1877–89.
82. Matson V, Fessler J, Bao R, et al. The commensal microbiome is associated with anti–PD-1 efficacy in metastatic melanoma patients. Science 2018;359(6371): 104–8.
83. Routy B, Le Chatelier E, Derosa L, et al. Gut microbiome influences efficacy of PD-1–based immunotherapy against epithelial tumors. Science 2018; 359(6371):91–7.
84. Vétizou M, Pitt JM, Daillère R, et al. Anticancer immunotherapy by CTLA-4 blockade relies on the gut microbiota. Science 2015;350(6264):1079–84.
85. Daillere R, Vetizou M, Waldschmitt N, et al. Enterococcus hirae and Barnesiella intestinihominis facilitate Cyclophosphamide-induced therapeutic immunomodu-latory effects. Immunity 2016;45(4):931–43.

86. Sivan A, Corrales L, Hubert N, et al. Commensal *Bifidobacterium* promotes anti-tumor immunity and facilitates anti–PD-L1 efficacy. Science 2015;350(6264): 1084–9.

87. Zitvogel L, Ma Y, Raoult D, et al. The microbiome in cancer immunotherapy: diagnostic tools and therapeutic strategies. Science 2018;359(6382):1366–70.

88. Turnbaugh PJ, Ley RE, Mahowald MA, et al. An obesity-associated gut microbiome with increased capacity for energy harvest. Nature 2006;444(7122): 1027–31.

89. Le Chatelier E, Nielsen T, Qin J, et al. Richness of human gut microbiome correlates with metabolic markers. Nature 2013;500:541.

90. Ridaura VK, Faith JJ, Rey FE, et al. Gut microbiota from twins discordant for obesity modulate adiposity and metabolic phenotypes in mice. Science 2013; 341(6150). https://doi.org/10.1126/science.1241214.

91. Zeevi D, Korem T, Zmora N, et al. Personalized nutrition by prediction of glycemic responses. Cell 2015;163(5):1079–94.

92. Korem T, Zeevi D, Zmora N, et al. Bread affects clinical parameters and induces gut microbiome-associated personal glycemic responses. Cell Metab 2017; 25(6):1243–53.e5.

Effective Use of the Laboratory in the Management of Patients with Inflammatory Bowel Diseases

M. Nedim Ince, MD[a],*, David E. Elliott, MD, PhD[b]

KEYWORDS

- Inflammatory bowel disease • Crohn's disease • Ulcerative colitis
- Genetic screening • Serology • Laboratory monitoring

KEY POINTS

- Ideal monitoring of patients with IBD would involve routine screening for mucosal healing by repeat endoscopic procedures or radiologic imaging.
- Although laboratory tests are not ideal in assessing disease activity, they constitute a reasonable adjunct to clinical assessment, endoscopy, and radiology.
- Routine laboratory assessment prevents nutritional deficiencies, helps improve the efficacy of medical therapy, and prevents medication-related or infectious complications.

THE USE OF LABORATORY TESTS FOR DIAGNOSIS, CLASSIFICATION, AND PROGNOSIS OF INFLAMMATORY BOWEL DISEASE

The peak range for onset of either Crohn's disease or ulcerative colitis is 15 to 30 years of age. Both diseases are life-long and patients worry how having inflammatory bowel disease (IBD) will influence their lives. In many, their illness will be minimally symptomatic and easy to treat; however, in others, the disease will cause severe tissue damage and require expensive medications with significant adverse effects, and quite possibly extensive surgery. Patient's symptoms can correlate poorly with mucosal inflammation.[1] Furthermore, in up to 10% of cases, it can be hard to distinguish whether chronic

Disclose statement: This work was supported by Merit Awards from the Department of Veterans Affairs BX002906 (MNI) and BX002715 (DEE).
[a] Department of Internal Medicine, Division of Gastroenterology and Hepatology, University of Iowa, Carver College of Medicine, University of Iowa Hospitals and Clinics, 4546 JCP, 200 Hawkins Drive, Iowa City, IA 52242, USA; [b] Department of Internal Medicine, Division of Gastroenterology and Hepatology, University of Iowa, Carver College of Medicine, University of Iowa Hospitals and Clinics, 4607 JCP, 200 Hawkins Drive, Iowa City, IA 52242, USA
* Corresponding author.
E-mail address: m-nedim-ince@uiowa.edu

Gastroenterol Clin N Am 48 (2019) 237–258
https://doi.org/10.1016/j.gtc.2019.02.006
0889-8553/19/© 2019 Elsevier Inc. All rights reserved.

inflammation limited to the colon is due to Crohn's disease or ulcerative colitis; this condition is named indeterminate colitis or IBD unclassified.[2] Patients desire a clear diagnosis, accurate prognosis, and a tailored plan of treatment. Therefore, clinicians look for tools to help reliably inform their patients and make cogent treatment decisions. This need requires a thorough assessment of patient's well-being with laboratory tests—besides the clinical evaluation—and drives the search for potential genetic or serologic markers that have prognostic significance.

THE USE OF GENETIC TESTING FOR DIAGNOSIS, CLASSIFICATION, AND PROGNOSIS OF INFLAMMATORY BOWEL DISEASE

Crohn's disease and ulcerative colitis have undergone extensive evaluation to identify genetic contributions to disease expression and prognosis. Multiple genome-wide association studies (GWAS) and immunochip surveys have identified approximately 200 loci that alter risk for developing IBD.[3] These loci include genes whose products are involved in cytokine expression, intracellular signaling, innate immune responses, chemotaxis, microbial product detection, and autophagy. Many (~70%) of the genes identified to confer risk for IBD also confer risk for developing other immune-mediated diseases.[4] The first identified Crohn's disease gene was NOD2/Card15, which is involved in recognition of microbial peptidoglycan (muramyl dipeptide) and regulation of autophagy. NOD2 is expressed by small intestinal Paneth cells[5] involved in microbial defense, and mutations in NOD2 are associated with ileal Crohn's disease.[6] Although carriage of a NOD2 mutation increases the risk for developing Crohn's disease[7] (an increase of 2-fold for simple heterozygotes [one allele harbors a pathogenic mutation] and 7- to 9-fold for homozygotes [each allele harbors the same pathogenic mutation] or complex heterozygotes [each allele harbors a different pathogenic mutation]), 7.8% of healthy controls carry a NOD2 mutation,[8] and most patients with Crohn's disease have normal NOD2 genes. A meta-analysis of 49 retrospective studies corporately evaluating 8892 patients with Crohn's disease found that patients with 2 NOD2 mutations are at higher (41% increased) risk for a complicated disease course (development of intestinal strictures and/or fistula) as compared with patients without NOD2 mutations.[9] However, having one mutant allele lacked prognostic value in predicting disease course.

Most GWAS in patients with IBD are focused on patients and controls of European descent. Whereas many of the IBD loci, which were identified using European populations, are also found in other groups, some loci such as NOD2 and ATG16L1 are not associated with disease in other populations.[10,11] On the other hand, additional novel loci that confer risk become evident in GWAS of non-European populations.[10–12] Different loci seem to act independently to contribute to disease risk.[4] To date, GWAS has identified only a small proportion of the estimated heritability for Crohn's disease (<25%) and ulcerative colitis (~16%) in European populations.[4,13] Thus, many additional genes, some with only rare variations, or some with only a statistically minimal increase in conferred risk, contribute to disease causality.

Genetic studies have demonstrated the importance of specific inflammatory/immune regulatory circuits in IBD development. Through these studies it has become clear that "standard" IBD is a complex polygenic disease that results from a multitude of genetic and environmental interactions. Although some gene mutations (like those in NOD2) associate with a given phenotype, many people without apparent disease carry the same mutation. To date, genetic analysis has not provided insight into a patient's future disease course beyond that made available by clinical presentation. Therefore, genetic analysis of patients with IBD for prognosis is not recommended.[14]

An exception to this guidance is for patients with early onset (IBD developing before age 10) and very early onset (IBD developing before age 2) disease, who may have a monogenic basis for disease due to highly pathogenic disruption of an important gene involved in immune function—such as XIAP,[15] ADAM17,[16] FOXP3,[17] IL-10/IL-10R,[18] or others.[19] In these cases, it is critically important to identify the genetic cause to determine if patients may benefit from an intensive intervention such as bone marrow transplantation.[20]

THE USE OF SERUM BIOMARKERS IN DIAGNOSIS, CLASSIFICATION, AND PROGNOSIS OF INFLAMMATORY BOWEL DISEASE

Patients with IBD often develop antibodies against autologous cellular antigens and/or microbial products (**Table 1**,[21–23]). Development of these antibodies may reflect: (A) a baseline aberrant immune regulation, which gives rise to both disease and antibody development; (B) a baseline impairment of epithelial barrier function allowing exposure

Table 1
Serologic markers (antibodies) in IBD

Marker	Antibody Target	UC (%)	CD (%)	Healthy Controls (%)
Most commonly seen in ulcerative colitis				
Anti-pANCA	Atypical pANCA; DNase-sensitive perinuclear neutrophil cytoplasmic antigens/DNA bound lactoferrin	24–85	2–18	0–8
Anti-GAB	Goblet cell antigens	15–47	1.4–33	0
Anti-PR3-ANCA	Proteinase 3	6	0	0
Most commonly seen in Crohn's disease				
ASCA	*S. cerevisiae* phosphopeptidomannan	0–29	29–71	0–16
ALCA	Laminarin–laminaribioside carbohydrate	0–22	8–76	0–23
ACCA	Chitin–citobioside carbohydrate	0–45	8–52	0–33
AMCA	Mannan–mannobioside carbohydrate	0–36	12–67	0–33
Anti-OmpC	*Escherichia coli* outer membrane porin C	11–31	17–55	5–31
Anti-I2	*Pseudomonas fluorescens* I2 transcription factor	2–42	26–60	2–12
Anti-CBir1	*Clostridium subphylum* XIVa cluster flagellin	6–36	50–56	8
Anti-PAB	Exocrine pancreatic antigens	0–23	26–39	0–8
Anti-GP2	Glycoprotein in pancreatic acinar cell and intestinal M cells	19	3–45	1–8
Anti-CUZD1	Pancreatic CUB/zona pellucida-like domain-containing protein	9–25	6–22	
Anti-L	Laminin carbohydrates	3–15	11–26	1
Anti-C	Chitin carbohydrates	2–15	10–25	2
Anti-A4-Fla2	A4 bacteria flagellin 2	59	6	0
Anti-A4-Fla-X	A4 bacteria flagellin X	57	6	2
Anti-GM-CSF	Granulocyte-macrophage colony-stimulating factor	NR	NR	NR

Abbreviation: NR, not reported.

to luminal antigens, which then drives the disease as well as antibody formation; and/ or (C) the ongoing and extensive mucosal injury that occurs in IBD. Supporting the first 2 etiologies is the observation that unaffected first-degree relatives of patients with Crohn's disease more frequently express these antibodies than the general population.[24–26] Support for the third etiology is the well-documented observation that patients with Crohn's disease positive for these antibodies often have worse disease.[27,28]

Multiple investigators have evaluated the expression profiles of diverse antibodies to determine if they can be used to predict disease type or course. The most studied antibodies are antineutrophil cytoplasmic antibody, which stains neutrophils in an atypical perinuclear pattern (atypical pANCA) and is most often expressed by patients with ulcerative colitis, and anti-*Saccharomyces cerevisiae* antibody (ASCA), which is most often expressed by patients with Crohn's disease. A meta-analysis of 60 studies corporately evaluating 7860 well-defined patients with IBD found that ANCA positivity had a sensitivity of 58% and a specificity of 88.5% for ulcerative colitis. Sensitivity and specificity were improved in pediatric patients with a negative ASCA level to 70.3% and 93.4%, respectively. Serologic ASCA positivity with ANCA negativity had a sensitivity of 54.6% and specificity of 92.8% for Crohn's disease.[29] Low sensitivity limits the usefulness of ASCA and ANCA testing, because many patients with IBD do not develop these antibodies. Negative serology does not exclude active IBD. Furthermore, using the previously given sensitivities and specificities,[29] and an expected prevalence of IBD at ~1.2%,[30] the positive predictive values of a positive atypical pANCA (5.8%) or ASCA (8.4%) are far too low to be used as a screening test in unselected patients. Inclusion of other antibodies (see **Table 1**) can increase sensitivity or specificity to some degree.[21] Indeed, testing may be of value if a significant fraction of "normal" patients with positive serology go on to develop IBD over time. A study from Israel has tested this in a cohort of serum repository samples that includes routine serum samples from armed forces enlistees. Baseline sera samples were positive for ASCA in 31.3% of 32 individuals who eventually developed Crohn's disease, and were positive for ANCA in 25% of 8 individuals who developed ulcerative colitis.[31] A similar study was performed using blood samples from 354,398 European volunteers, of whom 77 developed Crohn's disease and 167 developed ulcerative colitis.[32] That study found that 39% of the patients with Crohn's disease and 35% of the patients with ulcerative colitis had previous positive serology. The likelihood of positive serology was highest for those who developed IBD within 2.5 (Crohn's disease) or 2.9 (ulcerative colitis) years after the blood sample was taken. This suggests that many of these patients with IBD had subclinical disease at baseline driving their seropositivity. Using their test receiver operating characteristics (ROC) cutoffs, 10.4% of the case controls were seropositive for either Crohn's disease or ulcerative colitis markers. When applied to the whole volunteer population, for every seropositive patient identified within the follow-up period, 1227 and 623 individuals would have been considered at risk for Crohn's disease and ulcerative colitis, respectively. This confirms that these tests should not be used to screen for IBD in unselected groups.

Serologic tests have been evaluated to determine if they can differentiate which patients with indeterminate colitis will proceed to develop ulcerative colitis or Crohn's disease. A single-center observational study involving 117 patients with indeterminate colitis evaluated differential expression of atypical pANCA, ASCA, and anti-OmpC.[33] By 1 year after initial serology testing, the diagnosis of 50% enrollees had been reclassified as ulcerative colitis and 42% as Crohn's disease. Initial ANCA positivity had a 78% sensitivity and 44% specificity for predicting reclassification as ulcerative colitis. Initial ASCA positivity had an 18% sensitivity and 84% specificity for predicting reclassification as Crohn's disease. Anti-OmpC positivity fared no better, with a 27% sensitivity and 75% specificity for predicting reclassification as Crohn's disease. The investigators concluded that testing for these antibodies has limited use in predicting how indeterminate colitis will segregate.[33]

Serologic tests have been evaluated to determine if they can predict which patients will have a more complicated disease course. Patients with refractory ulcerative colitis require colectomy. Seropositivity with currently identified markers does not reliably predict which patients will need colectomy.[34,35] Following colectomy, many patients elect to have a surgically created ileoanal pouch rather than an ileostomy. Occasionally, this pouch becomes inflamed, a condition called pouchitis. It would benefit patients to know if they are at high risk for developing pouchitis and would be better served by electing to have an ileostomy. A meta-analysis of 14 studies corporately evaluating 335 patients with acute or chronic pouchitis found that the odds ratio for chronic pouchitis was 1.76 (CI, 1.19–2.61, $P < 0.01$) for patients with atypical pANCA positivity compared with those negative for that marker. Risk for chronic pouchitis was not associated with ASCA positivity. Neither serologic marker predicted development of acute pouchitis. Thus, testing for atypical pANCA, but not ASCA, is recommended for counseling of patients with ulcerative colitis considering ileoanal pouch surgery.[36]

Patients with severe Crohn's disease develop strictures and fistula that can require surgical excision of diseased bowel. Serologic tests have been evaluated to determine if they can predict which patients with Crohn's disease will go on to have a severe course. Most of these studies are retrospective, examining banked sera from patients with well-defined disease. Multiple studies have shown that those patients who have more severe course (stricturing or fistulizing disease needing surgery) more often express antibodies against multiple bacterial products and higher titer of those antibodies compared with patients with more limited disease.[28,37,38] However, determining predictive power requires prospective studies. A single-center prospective study evaluated 86 newly diagnosed Norwegian patients with Crohn's disease followed for a median of 30 months (range 16–64 months) who were initially tested for ASCA, atypical pANCA, AMCA, ALCA, and ACCA seropositivity (markers are described in **Table 1**). They found no association between baseline antibody positivity and development of a severe Crohn's disease course.[34] A second multi-center prospective study evaluated the ability of serology to predict disease recurrence following surgery in 169 patients with Crohn's disease.[39] They found no association of disease recurrence with ASCA positivity, but that the odds ratio for disease recurrence within 18 months of surgery was 6.4 (95% CI, 1.16–34.9, P=0.034) for patients positive for multiple other antibodies (anti-OmpC, anti-CBir, anti-A4-Fla2, and anti-A4-Fla-X) compared with seronegative patients. Therefore, patients with Crohn's disease who express multiple marker antibodies may benefit from more intensive medical therapy following resection.

Serologic tests also have been evaluated to determine if they can predict which patients will respond to specific medications. A single-center study examined seropositivity for atypical pANCA, ASCA, and anti-OmpC on the response of 230 patients with ulcerative colitis to antitumor necrosis factor alpha (anti-TNF-α) treatment.[40] The investigators found that neither atypical pANCA nor ASCA positivity identified patients that had suboptimal responses to anti-TNF-α therapy. Ulcerative colitis patients who expressed anti-OmpC had worse response to anti-TNF-α (odds ratio = 0.14; 95% CI, 0.03–0.60). This finding awaits confirmation in prospective studies. A Swedish study examined seropositivity for ASCA on the response of 1348 patients with Crohn's disease to infliximab (anti-TNF-α) treatment.[41] ASCA positivity did not correlate with infliximab response. At this time, the serologic profile should not dictate treatment choices.

LABORATORY ASSAYS FOR THE ASSESSMENT OF PRECIPITATING FACTORS ASSOCIATED WITH DISEASE ACTIVATION

Although diagnostic assays have limited value in identifying patients with IBD, other laboratory tests routinely assist the caregivers in providing standard or optimal care to individuals with established disease. In patients with IBD with active disease, caregivers strive for the induction of remission, and, for patients in remission, providers watch for reactivation of disease (**Box 1**). In ~10% of cases of IBD, who present with an acute flare, stool studies are positive for an enteric pathogen and approximately half of these infections are caused by *Clostridium difficile*.[42] In these cases, the infection is treated as the precipitating factor of an acute IBD flare. Usually, the diagnosis of *C difficile* infection is established by verification of a toxin-producing strain in liquid stool, using either a technique of nucleic acid amplification, such as polymerase chain reaction (PCR) or an enzyme immunoassay, to detect *C difficile* toxin A or toxin B. Assays based on nucleic acid amplification are more sensitive than assays that detect free toxins of *C difficile*. Hence, positive results obtained by a nucleic acid amplification assay can also detect a carrier, besides those patients with active *C difficile* infection. Although this fact raises the question of whether we over-diagnose our patients with *C difficile* infection by using nucleic acid amplification assay,[43] initial retrospective studies on this question indicate that diagnosis of *C difficile* infection based on nucleic acid amplification can reduce mortality.[44] Stool culture is performed to detect other enteric pathogens associated with an acute flare of IBD.

Pathologic significance of cytomegalovirus (CMV) infection in patients with IBD remains an important subject of dispute.[45,46] Different laboratory tests are used to diagnose CMV colitis, which include histology with or without immunohistochemistry, PCR from tissues, or PCR from the serum.[47] Many of these tests remain to be standardized. In general, CMV reactivation is more common in patients with Crohn's disease and patients with ulcerative colitis who are unresponsive to steroids or biologics. Patients with refractory disease should be checked for CMV infection and—if a high density of infection is found in the colon—treated with antiviral agents.[45]

Gluten sensitivity can occur in patients with IBD and gluten consumption can trigger symptoms similar to an acute IBD flare. Patients with IBD can have mildly increased anti-tTG IgA antibodies[48] and not have celiac disease. Furthermore, endoscopy findings in the small intestine can be similar in patients with Crohn's disease and in patients with celiac disease. One way to determine if a patient with Crohn's disease may have concurrent celiac disease is to perform genetic testing. Only 0.5% of patients with celiac disease lack both HLA-DQ2 and HLA-DQ8 antigens.[49] With such a high negative predictive value of HLA testing, genetic analysis is helpful in ruling *out*

Box 1
Aspects of clinical management in patients with established IBD

1. Induction of remission

2. Maintenance of remission

3. Prevention and treatment of medication-related side effects

4. Prevention and treatment of nutritional deficiencies

5. Prevention and treatment of infectious complications

6. Prevention and treatment of other complications

celiac disease in patients with IBD with gluten sensitivity. However, genetic testing is not helpful for ruling *in* celiac disease.

Laboratory tests also help health care providers insure proper nutrition and effective use of medications. Because several of these medications are potent immune suppressors—predisposing patients to severe infectious complications—laboratory tests are routinely used to screen and diagnose infections. Therefore, we discuss here effective use of laboratory tests in each of these aspects of clinical management (see **Box 1**).

Laboratory Tests to Check the Disease Activity after Induction of Remission

Although clinical assessment of patients and endoscopy findings are essential to assess acute flare and evaluate response to therapy, laboratory studies are widely used together with clinical assessment. For example, C-reactive protein (CRP) is a circulating pentametric protein that is produced in the liver in response to inflammation and binds lysophosphatidylcholine. Measurements of CRP or hypersensitive CRP are widely applied as indicators of acute phase inflammatory response including patients with IBD. High serum levels of CRP have been found to be associated with acute flare and normal levels correlate with remission. Furthermore, an increased CRP level predicts relapse after withdrawing immune modulatory medications.[50] In order for a biomarker to be reliable, it must be consistently high in patients with active disease and low or normal in patients in remission. Although high CRP level correlates well with active disease, normal CRP level may not reliably indicate remission.[51] This false-negative result associated with a lack of increased CRP level during flare may be influenced by a given patient's CRP genotype.[52] Hence, CRP measurement constitutes only an adjunct to clinical assessment of IBD activity rather than a test to replace clinical, endoscopic, and radiologic findings.[53] We measure CRP routinely in patients with IBD with fistulizing Crohn's disease, because an increase in CRP in these patients potentially indicates new abscess, bacteremia, or sepsis.[54] Erythrocyte sedimentation rate (ESR) can be used similarly to CRP to assess patients with IBD. Nonetheless, increased CRP level or ESR can be independently associated with age or sex.[55] Because of this, age-adjusted adaptation to calculate normal ESR has been proposed in the past.[56] Overall, endoscopic disease activity is found to correlate better with serum CRP level than with ESR.[57] An increase in blood platelet, white blood cell, or polymorphonuclear cell count also indicates an acute phase response. Therefore, a high platelet, white blood, or polymorphonuclear cell count can be used as an adjunct test to determine acute flare and the response to treatment. Mean platelet volume is an indicator of platelet turnover, and inversely correlates with IBD disease activity.[58] In addition, active IBD is associated with a hypercoagulable milieu and predisposes to thromboembolic complications. Although platelet count has been explored as an indicator of thromboembolic complications, no strong association has been found so far.[59] Antiplatelet agents have been suggested to be used in IBD to prevent thromboembolic complications. Because IBD is associated with bleeding from the gastrointestinal tract and that antiplatelet agents can increase the bleeding, and because nonsteroidal anti-inflammatory drugs can aggravate a flare of IBD, no consensus has been established in using antiplatelet agents to prevent thromboembolic complications in IBD. Furthermore, no consensus has been established in using platelet count and morphology as a routine indicator of IBD disease activity. These recommendations are different for inpatients admitted for medical therapy or surgery: hospitalized patients with IBD with moderate to severe disease and without severe bleeding should receive prophylaxis against development of deep vein thrombosis using low-dose unfractionated heparin, whereas patients with severe bleeding should have mechanical deep vein thrombosis prophylaxis using intermittent pneumatic compression.[60]

Fecal Markers Used in Diagnosis and Follow-Up of Intestinal Inflammation

Calprotectin has been the most investigated fecal marker of inflammation, although other markers have also been studied in laboratory assessment of intestinal inflammatory activity.[61] These include other cytoplasmic proteins of neutrophils, such as lactoferrin, S100A12, polymorphonuclear elastase, and M2-PK, an isoform of pyruvate kinase made by rapidly dividing cells.[62]

Calprotectin is the most abundant protein in the cytosol of neutrophils. It has also been found in lesser quantities in monocytes and macrophages. Calprotectin concentration is believed to increase in stool after inflammatory cells migrate to the intestine and—in the leaky environment of an inflamed gut—move into intestinal lumen to be excreted in the feces. The several-day stability of calprotectin in stool has made it an attractive candidate of noninvasive assessment for intestinal inflammation. Fecal calprotectin levels correlate well with endoscopic disease activity or CRP levels.[61] Calprotectin is now included in noninvasive routine assessment of IBD activity.

Treatment of flare with steroids, 5-aminosalicylates, immune modulators, or biologics aims for mucosal healing. The gold standard to assess for mucosal healing is repeating the endoscopy or colonoscopy, but this is a costly and invasive procedure in clinical practice. Measurement of stool calprotectin concentration has been found to correlate with endoscopic disease activity and is being used to monitor response to medical therapy. Calprotectin has also been suggested to be a useful marker to predict relapse.[61] This is also true for prediction of relapse after surgery in patients undergoing resection. Despite this strong evidence, it is important to remember that calprotectin is an indicator for inflammatory activity and leakage of neutrophils and their products into the stool in different conditions, such as infectious enteritis, diverticulitis, or even colorectal cancer. This property of being an indicator of inflammation or leakage of neutrophils into feces decreases the specificity of calprotectin in diagnosis of IBD, if the clinician has to differentiate between different inflammatory conditions, although it still can be used to differentiate between inflammatory and noninflammatory conditions, such as irritable bowel syndrome.[63]

Laboratory Tests to Check the Disease Activity During Maintenance of Remission

Laboratory tests to check for inflammatory activity during maintenance of remission are the same as those laboratory tests ordered during remission induction. Besides assessing for disease activity by clinical parameters, such as number of bowel movements, endoscopy, small bowel imaging or colonoscopy, blood or stool tests detailed above can be used to help with the overall assessment of the patient.

Additional laboratory tests are used during the maintenance of remission to evaluate the response to medical therapy. In most IBD cases with moderate to severe disease, medical therapy consists of an immune modulator, a biologic, or a combination of these 2 groups of medications. Azathioprine, 6-mercaptopurine, and methotrexate are frequently used as immune modulators and steroid sparing agents. These agents have a narrow therapeutic window and broad adverse effect profile, so close laboratory monitoring is needed for patients who are on immune modulators to prevent complications.

MONITORING THE EFFECTS OF MEDICATIONS, PREVENTION, AND TREATMENT OF SIDE EFFECTS OF MEDICATIONS
Laboratory Tests Routinely Used in Patients on Azathioprine and 6-Meraptopurine

After oral ingestion and absorption through the intestinal mucosa, azathioprine is metabolized into 6-mercaptopurine. This conversion can occur nonenzymatically, but the bulk is likely catalyzed by hepatic glutathione-S-transferases.[64] Subsequently, 6-mercaptopurine is converted to 6-thiouric acid, to 6-methyl mercaptopurine (6-MMPN), or to 6-thiogunanine (6-TGN). 6-Thiogunanine is believed to be the cytoactive intracellular metabolite of the prodrugs, azathioprine or 6-mercaptopurine (**Fig. 1**). Intracellular 6-TGN acts as a purine antagonist, inhibiting DNA synthesis, thus T-cell proliferation, and results in immune suppression. Azathioprine is prescribed at 2 to 3 mg/kg and 6-mercaptopurine at 1.0 to 1.5 mg/kg daily dose and the therapeutic efficacy of both medications correlates with intracellular concentration of 6-TGN. Intracellular concentration of 6-TGN is measured in erythrocytes and a concentration of 235 to 450 pmol/8 $\times$ 10^8 erythrocytes correlates with better therapeutic efficacy.[64]

Although response to treatment with azathioprine or 6-mercaptopurine is more frequently assessed by reviewing the patients' symptoms, endoscopic, or radiologic findings, 6-TGN concentration is often used, when remission is not induced or maintained and before making a decision to change the dose of the medication, change to a different immune modulator, or change to or add a biologic to the regimen. Also, increased intracellular concentrations of 6-TGN are associated with a risk of myelosuppression.[64] In patients with findings of myelosuppression, measuring 6-TGN concentration can help the provider better titrate the therapy. Hence, measuring 6-TGN can help the caregivers optimize the treatment with immune modulators, although azathioprine or 6-mercaptopurine are initially prescribed based on the patient's weight. Routine measurement of azathioprine metabolites is not recommended.[65]

6-Methyl mercaptopurine is another metabolite of azathioprine and 6-mercaptopurine. A high intracellular concentration of 6-MMPN or a high ratio of 6-MMPN to 6-TGN was found to be associated with poor response to treatment with azathioprine or 6-mercaptopurine.[66] Furthermore, a high intracellular concentration of 6-MMPN (>5700 pmol/8 $\times$ 10^8 erythrocytes) is associated with hepatotoxicity. Nevertheless, many patients with high red blood cell concentrations of 6-MMPN do not show any sign of hepatotoxicity, in this circumstance dose can continue with continued close monitoring of transaminases. However, if there is high red blood cell 6-MMPN

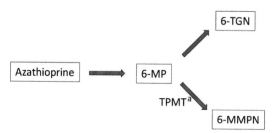

Fig. 1. Simplified scheme of azathioprine metabolism. Azathioprine is metabolized to 6-MP. 6-MP is then converted to 6-MMPN and 6-TGN. Each arrow in the graph can involve multiple steps or intermediates involved in the biochemical pathway associated with azathioprine and 6-MP metabolism. Other degradation products of 6-MP, such as 6-thiouric acid, are not shown for simplification purposes. [a] TPMT is involved in different pathways of 6-MP metabolism beside the conversion to 6-MMPN. These other pathways or intermediates are not shown for simplification.

concentrations, evidence of hepatotoxicity or ongoing clinical activity and low 6-TGN, adding allopurinol can shift the metabolism of azathioprine or 6-mercaptopurine from 6-MMP to 6-TGN to help optimize treatment with immune modulators.[67] Rarely, allopurinol can elicit life-threatening severe cutaneous adverse reactions. Development of severe cutaneous adverse reactions is strongly associated with HLA-B*5801 carriage in patients of Han Chinese, Korean, or Thai descent. Therefore, screening for that allele is warranted before starting allopurinol in patients with those ancestries. Investigation of a different treatment approach found that split dose azathioprine is associated with normalization of 6-MMPN levels and improvement of hepatotoxicity.[68]

Azathioprine or 6-MP is metabolized by the enzyme thiopurine methyl transferase (TPMT). If an individual has genetic deficiency of TPMT, the metabolites of the medications can accumulate to toxic levels and cause life-threatening leukopenia. Therefore, guidelines recommend to screen patients for TPMT enzyme activity before starting therapy, and avoid the use of azathioprine or 6-MP in patients who have low TPMT enzyme activity. Ninety percent of people have normal TPMT enzyme activity. Intermediate level of enzyme activity is seen in 9.7% of the population, and only 0.3% of people have 2 mutant alleles of TPMT and very low enzyme activity. Leukopenia is most frequently observed in patients with normal TPMT activity,[69] and therefore azathioprine and 6-MP should be used with caution in everyone. Severe leukopenia is most frequently observed in patients in the first 4 months after starting therapy. Many gastroenterologists start azathioprine or 6-MP at a subtherapeutic dose and increase the dose gradually, checking the patient's white cell count with differential frequently. The major reason why patients stop taking azathioprine or 6-MP is nausea and vomiting. Nausea and vomiting can subside in some patients if the medication is started at a low dose and the dose increased gradually. Yet, such dose escalation delays time to reach therapeutic levels, and studies show that it is safe to initiate thiopurine at full dose in patients with normal TPMT, as long as they are closely monitored.[70] Use of thiopurine requires initial frequent laboratory monitoring of transaminases, alkaline phosphatase, white cell count, and automated differential. Guidelines also recommend checking for white cell differential and transaminases every 3 months in the long term, because these adverse effects can occur anytime.

Laboratory Tests Routinely Used in Patients on Methotrexate

Methotrexate is an inhibitor of the enzyme dihydrofolate reductase and through this mechanism, methotrexate inhibits multiple pathways involved with inflammation.[71] Separate from dihydrofolate reductase inhibition, MTX may also inhibit JAK2/Stat5 signaling.[72] Methotrexate is effective in treating patients with Crohn's disease, if used parenterally at 15 to 25 mg per week.[73,74] It causes myelosuppression, especially if used together with other antifolate agents, such as trimethoprim-sulfamethoxazole. Bone marrow suppression should be carefully monitored in patients on methotrexate by checking complete blood count every 2 to 3 months. Often this side effect is reversible and blood counts normalize after stopping methotrexate. Yearly testing for folic acid level is recommended in pediatric patients with IBD.[75] Methotrexate-related cytopenias and other side effects—such as stomatitis—are reduced dramatically by concurrent use of folic acid.

Methotrexate is also hepatotoxic and liver tests should be monitored every 2 to 3 months, similar to performing complete blood counts. Methotrexate causes steatosis, stimulates stellate cells, and can contribute to hepatic fibrosis. Concurrent use of folic acid 1 mg per day or leucovorin 2.5 mg per week reduces the incidence of transaminitis.[76] Nevertheless, transaminase levels do not predict the development of hepatic fibrosis or cirrhosis and—in the past—liver biopsy was recommended after

1.5 g of cumulative dose and after every additional 1-g dose of methotrexate to monitor for progression of liver disease. Fortunately, moderate or severe hepatic fibrosis is rare in patients with Crohn's disease treated with methotrexate, and current protocols address measuring fibrosis noninvasively, for example, by transient elastography (FibroScan) and perform a liver biopsy only in those cases where the elastography shows significant fibrosis.[77] Clinical trials are underway to demonstrate whether such an approach will enable noninvasive assessment for hepatic fibrosis in patients with IBD on long-term use of methotrexate.

Laboratory Tests Routinely Used in Patients on Biologics

"Biologics" are monoclonal antibodies used in the treatment of patients with IBD with moderate to severe disease, as a monotherapy, or in combination with immune modulators. Three groups of biologics are approved for the treatment of patients with IBD. They are classified based on the endogenous inflammatory mediator they target. The first group are agents that target TNF-α: infliximab (Remicade, Inflectra, Renflexis, Ixifi), adalimumab (Humira, Amjevita, Cyltezo), certolizumab (Cimzia), and golimumab (Simponi). The second group are agents that target integrins used by inflammatory cells to access the intestine; vedolizumab (Entyvio, which targets integrin $\alpha4\beta7$) and natalizumab (Tysabri, which targets integrin $\alpha4$). The third group are agents that target interleukin-12 and/or interleukin-23: ustekinumab (Stelera).

Biologics are potent suppressors of targeted immune system function and some predispose patients to severe infections, such as tuberculosis. Furthermore, they are associated with toxicities to various organs.[78,79] Routine laboratory assessment is essential in patients with IBD before and during the treatment with biologics to monitor drug-related toxicities and to prevent or diagnose infectious complications in a timely manner. Biologics can be regarded as foreign proteins by the human immune system and these agents can trigger various forms of allergic or immune reactions. Concentration of the biologic agent in blood correlates with better response to the medication and, therefore, used by clinicians in the assessment of clinical response.[80] Recommended trough levels of biologics are discussed elsewhere.[65] Thus, caregivers use laboratory tests for various reasons in patients with IBD. Screening and diagnostic work-up for infections will be discussed in a later section.

Hematologic Complications of Biologic Agents

Use of biologics is frequently associated with mild and transient leukopenia. Leukopenia is usually associated with mild neutropenia and rarely necessitates stopping the medication. Biologics are very rarely associated with severe leukopenia, agranulocytosis, or pancytopenia.[81] It is recommended to screen patients with IBD on biologics routinely (ie, every 3–4 months) for complete blood counts with differential.

The Effects of Biologics on the Liver

Transient increase of transaminases or increase of cholestatic enzymes are common in patients on biologics.[82] If patients demonstrate mildly increased liver tests ($\leq$3-fold normal), monitor their liver tests every 2 weeks for 8 weeks or until the liver enzyme abnormalities subside. If the liver enzyme abnormalities are more than 3-fold, then a thorough work-up for hepatocellular disease should be initiated. This work-up should include evaluation for viral, metabolic, or autoimmune liver disease, abdominal ultrasound, and consideration of a liver biopsy.

Hepatitis serologies against hepatitis A virus (HAV), hepatitis B virus (HBV) and hepatitis C virus (HCV) are usually measured before starting therapy with a biologic and if not performed beforehand should be checked after liver enzymes are found high.

Serologic work-up for HBV infection should include the work-up for possible low level infection with HBV, as discussed below.

For patients with significantly increased transaminases, we routinely measure ceruloplasmin, alpha1-antitrypsin, and iron parameters when we assess for potential metabolic liver disease. Autoimmune hepatitis is usually associated with an increased serum IgG level and autoantibodies, such as antinuclear antibody, anti-smooth muscle antibody, anti-liver-kidney microsomes-1 (anti-LKM1), antimitochondrial antibody and perinuclear antinuclear cytoplasmic antibody (pANCA).[83] Drug-induced liver injury—in this case related to biologics—presents with eosinophilia and can display some features of autoimmune liver disease.[84] In cases of suspected autoimmune hepatitis, a liver biopsy should be performed.

Therapeutic Monitoring of Biologics (Trough Level of the Biologic Agent and Antibodies Against the Biologics)

Patients with IBD can lose response to the biologic agent. Although the mechanism of loss of response is not well-defined, 2 pharmacologic mechanisms have been proposed to cause loss of response to the biologic. These mechanisms are development of antibodies against the biologic agent and fluctuation in the trough level of the biologic due to altered metabolism.

Several clinical studies addressed the question whether antibodies against biologics are associated with loss of response to medication and affect the outcome of therapy. The results of these studies have shown that antibody formation against biologics puts the patient under risk for loss of response.[85,86] Furthermore, antibodies against biologics have been associated with allergic drug reactions. Drug reactions, including drug-induced lupus are discussed below.

Therapeutic trough level of anti-TNF-α agents correlates with mucosal healing and better long-term response to biologic therapy. Measuring trough levels in patients with primary unresponsiveness to biologic or secondary loss of response help the caregiver in making the decision to increase the dose of the biologic.[87] Measurement in other clinical scenarios, such as routine monitoring of trough levels in patients with clinical remission is less clear and not recommended.[65]

Drug-Induced Lupus

A severe complication of treatment with anti-TNFα agents is drug-induced lupus erythematous (ATIL).[88,89] It is characterized by muscle pain, skin lesions, and in severe cases can cause arthritis unresponsive to steroids, pleuritis, and pericarditis. Much of the time, muscle pain and rash after infusion or injection of the biologic are not due to a lupoid reaction and can be treated with antihistamines or a short course of steroids. Anti-TNF-α-induced lupus erythematosus should be considered in patients, whose symptoms are more severe and do not improve with a short course of antihistamines or steroids. The typical serology of ATIL is positive antinuclear antibody, positive antibody test against double-stranded DNA, and variable antihistone antibody positivity.[88,89] This is in contrast to classic drug-induced lupus erythematosus, which is antihistone antibody-positive and double-stranded DNA-negative. Besides these typical cases, atypical antibody parameters are frequently observed in patients with IBD who develop infusion/injection reaction to the biologics. In these atypical cases, we recommend trying a course of treatment of serum sickness, such as a course of antihistamines or steroids and—in patients who do not improve on this regimen—refer the patient to a rheumatologist for further evaluation.

Anti-TNF-α-induced lupus erythematosus is caused by antibodies that form against the Fc portion of the biologic. Certolizumab does not contain an Fc portion and therefore seems safe to be used in patients who develop ATIL after infliximab or adalimumab.[90] Vedolizumab is rarely associated with drug-induced lupus.[91,92]

Laboratory Tests Routinely Used in Patients on 5-Aminosalicylates

Various compounds with a 5-aminosalicylate active group are used to treat ulcerative colitis. The significant adverse effect profile of these agents is minimal in comparison with immune modulators or biologics. Among those, sulfasalazine can cause folic acid deficiency (discussed below). Otherwise, 5-aminosalicylates are associated with mild interstitial injury to the kidney and crystalluria.[93] Because these mild injuries rarely result in kidney insufficiency, current guidelines recommend yearly screening for blood urea nitrogen and creatinine.

Laboratory Tests Routinely Used in Patients Administered Cyclosporin

Cyclosporin is another agent used in steroid-refractory ulcerative colitis. This treatment should only be given to induce remission and to bridge to another agent—such as an immune modulator or vedolizumab—for the long-term maintenance of disease remission.[94,95] Cyclosporin therapy is started parenterally and—after seeing a clinical response—it is changed to oral form. Blood cyclosporin level should be checked frequently (every few days) and the dose of the medication should be adjusted to achieve a blood level of cyclosporin between 200 and 350 ng/mL. Patients on cyclosporin should be checked frequently for electrolyte abnormalities or renal toxicity. Hypomagnesemia or hypocholesterolemia raises seizure risk in patients on cyclosporin. Hypomagnesemia should be corrected or, in the case of hypocholesterolemia, the dose of cyclosporin should be adjusted to help prevent seizures in these individuals.

Laboratory Tests Routinely Used in Patients to Prevent or Treat Nutritional Deficiencies

Prevention and treatment of nutritional deficiencies in an IBD patient is important for the maintenance of health and to prevent complications related to deficiency of the specific factor. Patients with IBD with disease involvement of the terminal ileum frequently develop deficiency of vitamin B12. Patients on sulfasalazine and methotrexate are prone to folic acid deficiency. Patients with IBD can suffer from anemia due to depletion of iron stores (caused by chronic bleeding and malabsorption) or inability to use sufficient iron stores (anemia of chronic disease caused by ongoing inflammation). Vitamin D deficiency can also adversely affect the health of patients with IBD.

Vitamin B12 Deficiency

Vitamin B12 (cobalamin) is not produced by the human body but rather is absorbed from the diet. After food is ingested, hydrochloric acid and pepsin in the stomach separate vitamin B12 from its binding protein. This event leaves vitamin B12 free to dimerize with intrinsic factor, a protein that is produced by parietal cells of the stomach and required for the absorption of the vitamin in the terminal ileum.

Patients with IBD are prone to develop vitamin B12 deficiency, if they have terminal ileitis or have undergone ileal resection.[96] In the latter case, the length of resected ileum is a critical determinant for the development of pernicious anemia. Patients with IBD can also develop vitamin B12 deficiency as a consequence of small intestinal bacterial overgrowth.[97] Vitamin B12 deficiency causes megaloblastic anemia, progressive neurologic abnormalities, and cognitive problems. Therefore, it needs to be diagnosed in a timely manner and corrected. We routinely screen for vitamin B12 deficiency in our patients with IBD with ongoing or history of terminal ileal disease, history of terminal ileal resection or at risk for small intestinal bacterial overgrowth, and replace vitamin B12 orally or parenterally. Furthermore, we screen all patients with anemia or macrocytosis for vitamin B12 deficiency as part of the diagnostic workup. Last but not the least, it is important to remember that patients with ulcerative colitis can also develop vitamin B12 deficiency due to atrophic gastritis.[96]

Folic Acid Deficiency

Folic acid is produced by intestinal microbiota but is also provided through the diet. It is absorbed in the duodenum and proximal jejunum. Folate deficiency results in patients with IBD secondary to medication interactions, malabsorption, or inadequate nutrient intake.[98] Worldwide, the rate of folic acid deficiency began to decrease when it became policy to enrich several common nutrients for folic acid.[99] Although folic acid is absorbed in proximal small intestine, Crohn's disease affecting the distal small bowel or history of ileal resection are risk factors for folic acid deficiency and these findings suggest that small bowel malabsorption can be more diffuse than anticipated in these patients and that folic acid levels should be routinely checked and supplemented if deficient.[100] Two medications used frequently in the treatment of IBD, sulfasalazine and methotrexate, cause or worsen folic acid deficiency. Folic acid deficiency causes megaloblastic anemia, angular stomatitis, and depression. Although deficiency of folic acid—such as the deficiency of vitamin B12—increases the blood level of homocysteine, which is a risk factor for cardiovascular disease, several studies so far have failed to demonstrate a link between homocysteine level and venous or arterial thromboembolism in patients with IBD.[101] Folic acid levels are recommended to be checked yearly in patients with IBD on sulfasalazine or methotrexate.[75] Folic acid levels should also be measured in patients with IBD who are pregnant or are planning to become pregnant because folic acid deficiency in the first trimester predisposes to neural tube defects. Although folic acid level in blood is a good measure of folic acid supplies, measuring folic acid in red blood cells reflects the folic acid supplies over a period of 3 months and is therefore preferred.[98]

Iron Deficiency

Iron deficiency is the leading cause of anemia in patients with IBD.[98,102] The major etiology of iron deficiency in the context of this disease is chronic gastrointestinal blood loss. Chronic inflammation in IBD also interferes with use of iron by sequestering the mineral in monocytes and macrophages (anemia of chronic disease). Iron is absorbed in proximal small bowel, but iron deficiency secondary to severe IBD affecting the proximal small bowel is rare. Iron stores are assessed by quantitating serum iron, transferrin, iron binding capacity, and ferritin. Ferritin level can be misleading in a patient with a chronic inflammatory condition because ferritin is also an acute phase reactant and is expected to be high in a patient with active IBD. To differentiate between anemia of chronic disease and iron deficiency, clinicians also check the soluble transferrin receptor concentration in serum, which is elevated in iron deficiency but remains normal in anemia of chronic disease without iron deficiency. In light of this consideration, a group of experts has proposed guidelines toward correctly assessing the iron stores in patients with active IBD. These guidelines take into consideration the patient's symptoms and CRP level, beside the iron parameters, and use different cut-off values for ferritin in patients with or without active IBD.[103,104] If a patient has active disease, the cut-off value of ferritin is less than 100 ng/mL and for patients in remission the cut-off value is 30 ng/mL.[102] Although clinical induction of remission will reduce blood loss from the gastrointestinal tract, improve the absorption of nutrients, and is expected to improve the iron balance, iron deficiency causes severe fatigue and decreases the quality of life of patients. Therefore, assessment of iron parameters and aggressively correcting deficiency is recommended.[102]

Calcium and Vitamin D

Bone health is critical in patients with IBD because malnutrition, malabsorption, inflammation, and steroid use predispose to osteopenia.[105] Smoking is another risk factor for osteopenia and poor response to medical therapy. Although patients with IBD are prone to have a negative calcium balance because of poor intake due to factors such as lactose intolerance, intestinal losses in the setting of diarrhea, poor absorption related to steroid use or concomitant vitamin D deficiency, they rarely display hypocalcemia. Daily calcium intake in the amount of 1000 mg should be encouraged in these patients, although blood calcium levels are not assessed routinely. Vitamin D is critical to proper calcium homeostasis. In patients with IBD, low vitamin D levels are associated with increased disease activity and clinical relapse.[106] Prospective trials, which addressed the effect of vitamin D replacement on the course of IBD, have not shown a clear benefit so far.[106] Nonetheless, these studies overall have included a mixed population of patients with low or normal levels of vitamin D. As shown in patients with low vitamin D—evaluated longitudinally and retrospectively—frequent monitoring and replacement of vitamin D can have a benefit on the course of IBD.[107] Furthermore, it has been proposed that vitamin D replacement can prevent colorectal cancer associated with long standing colitis in patients with IBD.[108] Therefore, vitamin D should be checked yearly and if deficient replaced.

Prevention and Treatment of Infectious Complications

Patients with IBD and on immune modulators or biologics are prone to develop an aggressive course of hepatitis, tuberculosis, or fungal infections, such as histoplasmosis.

Patients are routinely screened for HAV, HBV, and HCV, and vaccinated against HAV and HBV if they are seronegative. Patients who are seropositive against HAV or HBV can be immune against these viruses by vaccination or after natural infection. In this context, a positive serology against HBV core antigen (anti-HBc) besides a positive serology against HBV surface antigen (anti-HBs) suggests immunity against natural infection, whereas a negative anti-HBc result with a positive anti-HBs result suggests immunity after vaccination. Patients who cleared HBV after natural infection can have ongoing replication of HBV in immune privileged sites without causing systemic recurrence of HBV infection.[109,110] Therefore, patients undergoing high-risk immune suppressive therapy with chemotherapeutic agents or rituximab can develop recurrence of HBV infection after cleared natural infection.[111] Although the relationship between immune suppression with biologics and the recurrence of HBV infection in anti-HBc-seropositive and anti-HBs-seropositive patients with IBD is less clear, it is recommended that HBV-DNA be routinely checked (for example every 3–6 months) in these individuals to diagnose active HBV infection in a timely manner.[112]

Reactivation of tuberculosis infection is a severe complication of treatment with some biologics.[113] Furthermore, patients with IBD are at risk to develop tuberculosis infection due to immune suppression secondary to use of steroids or immune modulatory agents. Therefore, it is important to diagnose patients with latent tuberculosis infection and treat them with anti-tuberculosis medications before or at the beginning of treatment with biologics, although it is unclear for now, whether such a strategy will eliminate the risk of reactivation.[114] Latent tuberculosis infection is diagnosed by a T-cell response against mycobacteria, either by an in vivo test that quantitates skin reaction to purified protein derivative (PPD) of mycobacteria (tuberculin skin test [TST]) or an in vitro interferon gamma release assay (IGRA). The sensitivity of PPD and IGRA are comparable, although IGRA is more specific, and is therefore preferred. The IGRA test can be affected by the booster effect after repeat PPD testing,[115] similar to a TST. Last, but not least, a PPD test or IGRA can be false-negative in an immune-suppressed patient. Patients with IBD are immune suppressed by the extent of inflammation, due to use of steroids, immune modulators, and biologics. Hence, diagnosing latent or active tuberculosis infection requires great care because of the potential high rate of false negativity. Some countries have included a chest radiograph in diagnostic protocols of latent tuberculosis infection to increase the diagnostic yield.[116] This can be a reasonable approach in populations where tuberculosis is prevalent.

Some clinicians advocate routine check of serology against measles, mumps and rubella in IBD patients. Although protection of patients against these infections is a concern - especially with rising incidence of measles in the United States - protection by vaccination requires the use of live vaccines and live vaccines can cause severe infection in immune suppressed individuals. Therefore, we prefer not to include measles, mumps and rubella serology in our routine laboratory work-up for now.

Diagnosis of infections in immune-suppressed patients with IBD requires great care and thorough work-up. We perform such a work-up together with specialists of infectious diseases. Laboratory tests of infectious complications and a thorough infection work-up in patients with IBD is beyond the scope of this article.

SUMMARY

Ideal monitoring of patients with IBD would involve routine screening for mucosal healing by repeat endoscopic procedures or radiologic imaging. Nonetheless, this is an impractical, costly approach in clinical routines, and each intervention carries risk. Although laboratory tests are not ideal in assessing disease activity, they constitute a reasonable adjunct to clinical assessment, endoscopy, and radiology. Furthermore, routine laboratory assessment prevents nutritional deficiencies, helps improve the efficacy of medical therapy, and prevents medication-related or infectious complications.

REFERENCES

1. Minderhoud IM, Samsom M, Oldenburg B. What predicts mucosal inflammation in Crohn's disease patients? Inflamm Bowel Dis 2007;13(12):1567–72.
2. Geboes K, De Hertogh G. Indeterminate colitis. Inflamm Bowel Dis 2003;9(5): 324–31.
3. Ye BD, McGovern DP. Genetic variation in IBD: progress, clues to pathogenesis and possible clinical utility. Expert Rev Clin Immunol 2016;12(10):1091–107.
4. Jostins L, Ripke S, Weersma RK, et al. Host-microbe interactions have shaped the genetic architecture of inflammatory bowel disease. Nature 2012;491(7422): 119–24.
5. Ogura Y, Lala S, Xin W, et al. Expression of NOD2 in Paneth cells: a possible link to Crohn's ileitis. Gut 2003;52(11):1591–7.
6. Cuthbert AP, Fisher SA, Mirza MM, et al. The contribution of NOD2 gene mutations to the risk and site of disease in inflammatory bowel disease. Gastroenterology 2002;122(4):867–74.
7. Yazdanyar S, Weischer M, Nordestgaard BG. Genotyping for NOD2 genetic variants and Crohn's disease: a metaanalysis. Clin Chem 2009;55(11):1950–7.

8. Hugot JP, Zaccaria I, Cavanaugh J, et al. Prevalence of CARD15/NOD2 mutations in Caucasian healthy people. Am J Gastroenterol 2007;102(6):1259–67.

9. Adler J, Rangwalla SC, Dwamena BA, et al. The prognostic power of the NOD2 genotype for complicated Crohn's disease: a meta-analysis. Am J Gastroenterol 2011;106(4):699–712.

10. Hirano A, Yamazaki K, Umeno J, et al. Association study of 71 European Crohn's disease susceptibility loci in a Japanese population. Inflamm Bowel Dis 2013; 19(3):526–33.

11. Yang SK, Hong M, Zhao W, et al. Genome-wide association study of Crohn's disease in Koreans revealed three new susceptibility loci and common attributes of genetic susceptibility across ethnic populations. Gut 2014;63(1):80–7.

12. Brant SR, Okou DT, Simpson CL, et al. Genome-wide association study identifies African-specific susceptibility loci in African Americans with inflammatory bowel disease. Gastroenterology 2017;152(1):206–17.e2.

13. Anderson CA, Boucher G, Lees CW, et al. Meta-analysis identifies 29 additional ulcerative colitis risk loci, increasing the number of confirmed associations to 47. Nat Genet 2011;43(3):246–52.

14. Boyapati RK, Kalla R, Satsangi J, et al. Biomarkers in search of precision medicine in IBD. Am J Gastroenterol 2016;111(12):1682–90.

15. Zeissig Y, Petersen BS, Milutinovic S, et al. XIAP variants in male Crohn's disease. Gut 2015;64(1):66–76.

16. Blaydon DC, Biancheri P, Di WL, et al. Inflammatory skin and bowel disease linked to ADAM17 deletion. N Engl J Med 2011;365(16):1502–8.

17. Okou DT, Mondal K, Faubion WA, et al. Exome sequencing identifies a novel FOXP3 mutation in a 2-generation family with inflammatory bowel disease. J Pediatr Gastroenterol Nutr 2014;58(5):561–8.

18. Pigneur B, Escher J, Elawad M, et al. Phenotypic characterization of very early-onset IBD due to mutations in the IL10, IL10 receptor alpha or beta gene: a survey of the Genius Working Group. Inflamm Bowel Dis 2013;19(13):2820–8.

19. Kammermeier J, Dziubak R, Pescarin M, et al. Phenotypic and genotypic characterisation of inflammatory bowel disease presenting before the age of 2 years. J Crohns Colitis 2017;11(1):60–9.

20. Murugan D, Albert MH, Langemeier J, et al. Very early onset inflammatory bowel disease associated with aberrant trafficking of IL-10R1 and cure by T cell replete haploidentical bone marrow transplantation. J Clin Immunol 2014;34(3):331–9.

21. Prideaux L, De Cruz P, Ng SC, et al. Serological antibodies in inflammatory bowel disease: a systematic review. Inflamm Bowel Dis 2012;18(7):1340–55.

22. Bonneau J, Dumestre-Perard C, Rinaudo-Gaujous M, et al. Systematic review: new serological markers (anti-glycan, anti-GP2, anti-GM-CSF Ab) in the prediction of IBD patient outcomes. Autoimmun Rev 2015;14(3):231–45.

23. Kuna AT. Serological markers of inflammatory bowel disease. Biochem Med (Zagreb) 2013;23(1):28–42.

24. Sendid B, Quinton JF, Charrier G, et al. Anti-*Saccharomyces cerevisiae* mannan antibodies in familial Crohn's disease. Am J Gastroenterol 1998;93(8):1306–10.

25. Seibold F, Stich O, Hufnagl R, et al. Anti-*Saccharomyces cerevisiae* antibodies in inflammatory bowel disease: a family study. Scand J Gastroenterol 2001; 36(2):196–201.

26. Kamm F, Strauch U, Degenhardt F, et al. Serum anti-glycan-antibodies in relatives of patients with inflammatory bowel disease. PLoS One 2018;13(3): e0194222.

27. Arnott ID, Landers CJ, Nimmo EJ, et al. Sero-reactivity to microbial components in Crohn's disease is associated with disease severity and progression, but not NOD2/CARD15 genotype. Am J Gastroenterol 2004;99(12):2376–84.

28. Schoepfer AM, Schaffer T, Mueller S, et al. Phenotypic associations of Crohn's disease with antibodies to flagellins A4-Fla2 and Fla-X, ASCA, p-ANCA, PAB, and NOD2 mutations in a Swiss Cohort. Inflamm Bowel Dis 2009;15(9):1358–67.

29. Reese GE, Constantinides VA, Simillis C, et al. Diagnostic precision of anti-*Saccharomyces cerevisiae* antibodies and perinuclear antineutrophil cytoplasmic antibodies in inflammatory bowel disease. Am J Gastroenterol 2006; 101(10):2410–22.

30. Dahlhamer JM, Zammitti EP, Ward BW, et al. Prevalence of inflammatory bowel disease among adults aged >/=18 years - United States, 2015. MMWR Morb Mortal Wkly Rep 2016;65(42):1166–9.

31. Israeli E, Grotto I, Gilburd B, et al. Anti-*Saccharomyces cerevisiae* and antineutrophil cytoplasmic antibodies as predictors of inflammatory bowel disease. Gut 2005;54(9):1232–6.

32. van Schaik FD, Oldenburg B, Hart AR, et al. Serological markers predict inflammatory bowel disease years before the diagnosis. Gut 2013;62(5):683–8.

33. Sura SP, Ahmed A, Cheifetz AS, et al. Characteristics of inflammatory bowel disease serology in patients with indeterminate colitis. J Clin Gastroenterol 2014; 48(4):351–5.

34. Smids C, Horjus Talabur Horje CS, Groenen MJM, et al. The value of serum antibodies in differentiating inflammatory bowel disease, predicting disease activity and disease course in the newly diagnosed patient. Scand J Gastroenterol 2017;52(10):1104–12.

35. Kovacs G, Sipeki N, Suga B, et al. Significance of serological markers in the disease course of ulcerative colitis in a prospective clinical cohort of patients. PLoS One 2018;13(3):e0194166.

36. Singh S, Sharma PK, Loftus EV Jr, et al. Meta-analysis: serological markers and the risk of acute and chronic pouchitis. Aliment Pharmacol Ther 2013;37(9): 867–75.

37. Dassopoulos T, Frangakis C, Cruz-Correa M, et al. Antibodies to *Saccharomyces cerevisiae* in Crohn's disease: higher titers are associated with a greater frequency of mutant NOD2/CARD15 alleles and with a higher probability of complicated disease. Inflamm Bowel Dis 2007;13(2):143–51.

38. Mow WS, Vasiliauskas EA, Lin YC, et al. Association of antibody responses to microbial antigens and complications of small bowel Crohn's disease. Gastroenterology 2004;126(2):414–24.

39. Hamilton AL, Kamm MA, De Cruz P, et al. Serologic antibodies in relation to outcome in postoperative Crohn's disease. J Gastroenterol Hepatol 2017; 32(6):1195–203.

40. Kevans D, Waterman M, Milgrom R, et al. Serological markers associated with disease behavior and response to anti-tumor necrosis factor therapy in ulcerative colitis. J Gastroenterol Hepatol 2015;30(1):64–70.

41. Lonnkvist MH, Befrits R, Lundberg JO, et al. Infliximab in clinical routine: experience with Crohn's disease and biomarkers of inflammation over 5 years. Eur J Gastroenterol Hepatol 2009;21(10):1168–76.

42. Mylonaki M, Langmead L, Pantes A, et al. Enteric infection in relapse of inflammatory bowel disease: importance of microbiological examination of stool. Eur J Gastroenterol Hepatol 2004;16(8):775–8.

43. Gateau C, Couturier J, Coia J, et al. How to: diagnose infection caused by *Clostridium difficile*. Clin Microbiol Infect 2018;24(5):463–8.
44. Avni T, Babich T, Ben-Zvi H, et al. Molecular-based diagnosis of *Clostridium difficile* infection is associated with reduced mortality. Eur J Clin Microbiol Infect Dis 2018;37(6):1137–42.
45. Pillet S, Pozzetto B, Roblin X. Cytomegalovirus and ulcerative colitis: place of antiviral therapy. World J Gastroenterol 2016;22(6):2030–45.
46. Johnson J, Affolter K, Boynton K, et al. CMV disease in IBD: comparison of diagnostic tests and correlation with disease outcome. Inflamm Bowel Dis 2018; 24(7):1539–46.
47. Romkens TE, Bulte GJ, Nissen LH, et al. Cytomegalovirus in inflammatory bowel disease: a systematic review. World J Gastroenterol 2016;22(3):1321–30.
48. Sardy M, Csikos M, Geisen C, et al. Tissue transglutaminase ELISA positivity in autoimmune disease independent of gluten-sensitive disease. Clin Chim Acta 2007;376(1–2):126–35.
49. Bosca-Watts MM, Minguez M, Planelles D, et al. HLA-DQ: celiac disease vs inflammatory bowel disease. World J Gastroenterol 2018;24(1):96–103.
50. Treton X, Bouhnik Y, Mary JY, et al, Groupe D'Etude Thérapeutique Des Affections Inflammatoires Du Tube Digestif (GETAID). Azathioprine withdrawal in patients with Crohn's disease maintained on prolonged remission: a high risk of relapse. Clin Gastroenterol Hepatol 2009;7(1):80–5.
51. Chang S, Malter L, Hudesman D. Disease monitoring in inflammatory bowel disease. World J Gastroenterol 2015;21(40):11246–59.
52. Moran CJ, Kaplan JL, Winter HS. Genetic variation affects C-reactive protein elevations in Crohn's disease. Inflamm Bowel Dis 2018. https://doi.org/10.1093/ibd/izy100.
53. Miranda-Garcia P, Chaparro M, Gisbert JP. Correlation between serological biomarkers and endoscopic activity in patients with inflammatory bowel disease. Gastroenterol Hepatol 2016;39(8):508–15.
54. Pettit SH, Holbrook IB, Irving MH. Comparison of clinical scores and acute phase proteins in the assessment of acute Crohn's disease. Br J Surg 1985; 72(12):1013–6.
55. Siemons L, Ten Klooster PM, Vonkeman HE, et al. How age and sex affect the erythrocyte sedimentation rate and C-reactive protein in early rheumatoid arthritis. BMC Musculoskelet Disord 2014;15:368.
56. Miller A, Green M, Robinson D. Simple rule for calculating normal erythrocyte sedimentation rate. Br Med J (Clin Res Ed) 1983;286(6361):266.
57. Vermeire S, Van Assche G, Rutgeerts P. Laboratory markers in IBD: useful, magic, or unnecessary toys? Gut 2006;55(3):426–31.
58. Kapsoritakis AN, Koukourakis MI, Sfiridaki A, et al. Mean platelet volume: a useful marker of inflammatory bowel disease activity. Am J Gastroenterol 2001; 96(3):776–81.
59. Voudoukis E, Karmiris K, Koutroubakis IE. Multipotent role of platelets in inflammatory bowel diseases: a clinical approach. World J Gastroenterol 2014;20(12): 3180–90.
60. Nguyen GC, Bernstein CN, Bitton A, et al. Consensus statements on the risk, prevention, and treatment of venous thromboembolism in inflammatory bowel disease: Canadian Association of Gastroenterology. Gastroenterology 2014; 146(3):835–48.e6.
61. Walsham NE, Sherwood RA. Fecal calprotectin in inflammatory bowel disease. Clin Exp Gastroenterol 2016;9:21–9.

62. Turner D, Leach ST, Mack D, et al. Faecal calprotectin, lactoferrin, M2-pyruvate kinase and S100A12 in severe ulcerative colitis: a prospective multicentre comparison of predicting outcomes and monitoring response. Gut 2010;59(9): 1207–12.

63. Menees SB, Powell C, Kurlander J, et al. A meta-analysis of the utility of C-reactive protein, erythrocyte sedimentation rate, fecal calprotectin, and fecal lactoferrin to exclude inflammatory bowel disease in adults with IBS. Am J Gastroenterol 2015;110(3):444–54.

64. Gearry RB, Barclay ML. Azathioprine and 6-mercaptopurine pharmacogenetics and metabolite monitoring in inflammatory bowel disease. J Gastroenterol Hepatol 2005;20(8):1149–57.

65. Feuerstein JD, Nguyen GC, Kupfer SS, et al, American Gastroenterological Association Institute Clinical Guidelines Committee. American Gastroenterological Association Institute Guideline on therapeutic drug monitoring in inflammatory bowel disease. Gastroenterology 2017;153(3):827–34.

66. Jharap B, Seinen ML, de Boer NK, et al. Thiopurine therapy in inflammatory bowel disease patients: analyses of two 8-year intercept cohorts. Inflamm Bowel Dis 2010;16(9):1541–9.

67. Friedman AB, Brown SJ, Bampton P, et al. Randomised clinical trial: efficacy, safety and dosage of adjunctive allopurinol in azathioprine/mercaptopurine nonresponders (AAA Study). Aliment Pharmacol Ther 2018;47(8):1092–102.

68. Shih DQ, Nguyen M, Zheng L, et al. Split-dose administration of thiopurine drugs: a novel and effective strategy for managing preferential 6-MMP metabolism. Aliment Pharmacol Ther 2012;36(5):449–58.

69. Colombel JF, Ferrari N, Debuysere H, et al. Genotypic analysis of thiopurine S-methyltransferase in patients with Crohn's disease and severe myelosuppression during azathioprine therapy. Gastroenterology 2000;118(6):1025–30.

70. Benmassaoud A, Xie X, AlYafi M, et al. Thiopurines in the management of Crohn's disease: safety and efficacy profile in patients with normal TPMT activity - a retrospective study. Can J Gastroenterol Hepatol 2016;2016:1034834.

71. Chan ES, Cronstein BN. Methotrexate–how does it really work? Nat Rev Rheumatol 2010;6(3):175–8.

72. Thomas S, Fisher KH, Snowden JA, et al. Methotrexate is a JAK/STAT pathway inhibitor. PLoS One 2015;10(7):e0130078.

73. Feagan BG, Rochon J, Fedorak RN, et al. Methotrexate for the treatment of Crohn's disease. The North American Crohn's Study Group Investigators. N Engl J Med 1995;332(5):292–7.

74. Patel V, Wang Y, MacDonald JK, et al. Methotrexate for maintenance of remission in Crohn's disease. Cochrane Database Syst Rev 2014;(8):CD006884.

75. Miele E, Shamir R, Aloi M, et al. Nutrition in pediatric inflammatory bowel disease: a position paper on behalf of the Porto Inflammatory Bowel Disease Group of the European Society of Pediatric Gastroenterology, Hepatology and Nutrition. J Pediatr Gastroenterol Nutr 2018;66(4):687–708.

76. Prey S, Paul C. Effect of folic or folinic acid supplementation on methotrexate-associated safety and efficacy in inflammatory disease: a systematic review. Br J Dermatol 2009;160(3):622–8.

77. Shamberg L, Vaziri H. Hepatotoxicity of inflammatory bowel disease medications. J Clin Gastroenterol 2018;52(8):674–84.

78. Reddy JG, Loftus EV Jr. Safety of infliximab and other biologic agents in the inflammatory bowel diseases. Gastroenterol Clin North Am 2006;35(4):837–55.

79. Stallmach A, Hagel S, Bruns T. Adverse effects of biologics used for treating IBD. Best Pract Res Clin Gastroenterol 2010;24(2):167–82.
80. Sheasgreen C, Nguyen GC. The evolving evidence for therapeutic drug monitoring of monoclonal antibodies in inflammatory bowel disease. Curr Gastroenterol Rep 2017;19(5):19.
81. Sebastian S, Ashton K, Houston Y, et al. Anti-TNF therapy induced immune neutropenia in Crohns disease - report of 2 cases and review of literature. J Crohns Colitis 2012;6(6):713–6.
82. Koller T, Galambosova M, Filakovska S, et al. Drug-induced liver injury in inflammatory bowel disease: 1-year prospective observational study. World J Gastroenterol 2017;23(22):4102–11.
83. Schmeltzer PA, Russo MW. Clinical narrative: autoimmune hepatitis. Am J Gastroenterol 2018;113(7):951–8.
84. Rodrigues S, Lopes S, Magro F, et al. Autoimmune hepatitis and anti-tumor necrosis factor alpha therapy: a single center report of 8 cases. World J Gastroenterol 2015;21(24):7584–8.
85. Ben-Horin S, Chowers Y. Review article: loss of response to anti-TNF treatments in Crohn's disease. Aliment Pharmacol Ther 2011;33(9):987–95.
86. Roda G, Jharap B, Neeraj N, et al. Loss of response to anti-TNFs: definition, epidemiology, and management. Clin Transl Gastroenterol 2016;7:e135.
87. Ben-Horin S, Kopylov U, Chowers Y. Optimizing anti-TNF treatments in inflammatory bowel disease. Autoimmun Rev 2014;13(1):24–30.
88. Williams EL, Gadola S, Edwards CJ. Anti-TNF-induced lupus. Rheumatology (Oxford) 2009;48(7):716–20.
89. Shovman O, Tamar S, Amital H, et al. Diverse patterns of anti-TNF-alpha-induced lupus: case series and review of the literature. Clin Rheumatol 2018;37(2):563–8.
90. Verma HD, Scherl EJ, Jacob VE, et al. Anti-nuclear antibody positivity and the use of certolizumab in inflammatory bowel disease patients who have had arthralgias or lupus-like reactions from infliximab or adalimumab. J Dig Dis 2011;12(5):379–83.
91. Sandborn WJ, Feagan BG, Rutgeerts P, et al. Vedolizumab as induction and maintenance therapy for Crohn's disease. N Engl J Med 2013;369(8):711–21.
92. Feagan BG, Rutgeerts P, Sands BE, et al. Vedolizumab as induction and maintenance therapy for ulcerative colitis. N Engl J Med 2013;369(8):699–710.
93. Siddique N, Farmer C, Muller AF. Do gastroenterologists monitor their patients taking 5-amino-salicylates following initiation of treatment. Frontline Gastroenterol 2015;6(1):27–31.
94. Bernstein CN, Kornbluth A. Yes, we are still talking about cylosporin vs. infliximab in steroid resistant acute severe ulcerative colitis. Am J Gastroenterol 2017;112(11):1719–21.
95. Christensen B, Gibson P, Micic D, et al. Safety and efficacy of combination treatment with calcineurin inhibitors and vedolizumab in patients with refractory inflammatory bowel disease. Clin Gastroenterol Hepatol 2019;17(3):486–93.
96. Ward MG, Kariyawasam VC, Mogan SB, et al. Prevalence and risk factors for functional vitamin B12 deficiency in patients with Crohn's disease. Inflamm Bowel Dis 2015;21(12):2839–47.
97. Greco A, Caviglia GP, Brignolo P, et al. Glucose breath test and Crohn's disease: diagnosis of small intestinal bacterial overgrowth and evaluation of therapeutic response. Scand J Gastroenterol 2015;50(11):1376–81.

98. Hwang C, Ross V, Mahadevan U. Micronutrient deficiencies in inflammatory bowel disease: from A to zinc. Inflamm Bowel Dis 2012;18(10):1961–81.

99. Crider KS, Bailey LB, Berry RJ. Folic acid food fortification - its history, effect, concerns, and future directions. Nutrients 2011;3(3):370–84.

100. Huang S, Ma J, Zhu M, et al. Status of serum vitamin B12 and folate in patients with inflammatory bowel disease in China. Intest Res 2017;15(1):103–8.

101. Oldenburg B, Fijnheer R, van der Griend R, et al. Homocysteine in inflammatory bowel disease: a risk factor for thromboembolic complications? Am J Gastroenterol 2000;95(10):2825–30.

102. Peyrin-Biroulet L, Lopez A, Cummings JRF, et al. Review article: treating-to-target for inflammatory bowel disease-associated anaemia. Aliment Pharmacol Ther 2018;48(6):610–7.

103. Gasche C, Berstad A, Befrits R, et al. Guidelines on the diagnosis and management of iron deficiency and anemia in inflammatory bowel diseases. Inflamm Bowel Dis 2007;13(12):1545–53.

104. Dignass AU, Gasche C, Bettenworth D, et al. European consensus on the diagnosis and management of iron deficiency and anaemia in inflammatory bowel diseases. J Crohns Colitis 2015;9(3):211–22.

105. Abegunde AT, Muhammad BH, Ali T. Preventive health measures in inflammatory bowel disease. World J Gastroenterol 2016;22(34):7625–44.

106. Gubatan J, Moss AC. Vitamin D in inflammatory bowel disease: more than just a supplement. Curr Opin Gastroenterol 2018;34(4):217–25.

107. Kabbani TA, Koutroubakis IE, Schoen RE, et al. Association of vitamin D level with clinical status in inflammatory bowel disease: a 5-year longitudinal study. Am J Gastroenterol 2016;111(5):712–9.

108. Meeker S, Seamons A, Maggio-Price L, et al. Protective links between vitamin D, inflammatory bowel disease and colon cancer. World J Gastroenterol 2016; 22(3):933–48.

109. Cacciola I, Pollicino T, Squadrito G, et al. Occult hepatitis B virus infection in patients with chronic hepatitis C liver disease. N Engl J Med 1999;341(1):22–6.

110. Wu T, Kwok RM, Tran TT. Isolated anti-HBc: the relevance of hepatitis B core antibody - A review of new issues. Am J Gastroenterol 2017;112(12):1780–8.

111. Seto WK, Chan TS, Hwang YY, et al. Hepatitis B reactivation in occult viral carriers undergoing hematopoietic stem cell transplantation: a prospective study. Hepatology 2017;65(5):1451–61.

112. Mori S, Fujiyama S. Hepatitis B virus reactivation associated with antirheumatic therapy: risk and prophylaxis recommendations. World J Gastroenterol 2015; 21(36):10274–89.

113. Jung SM, Ju JH, Park MS, et al. Risk of tuberculosis in patients treated with anti-tumor necrosis factor therapy: a nationwide study in South Korea, a country with an intermediate tuberculosis burden. Int J Rheum Dis 2015;18(3):323–30.

114. Ramos GP, Stroh G, Al-Bawardy B, et al. Outcomes of treatment for latent tuberculosis infection in patients with inflammatory bowel disease receiving biologic therapy. Inflamm Bowel Dis 2018;24(10):2272–7.

115. van Zyl-Smit RN, Zwerling A, Dheda K, et al. Within-subject variability of interferon-g assay results for tuberculosis and boosting effect of tuberculin skin testing: a systematic review. PLoS One 2009;4(12):e8517.

116. National Tuberculosis Advisory Committee. Position statement on interferon-gamma release assays in the detection of latent tuberculosis infection. Commun Dis Intell Q Rep 2012;36(1):125–31.

Laboratory Diagnosis and Monitoring of Viral Hepatitis

Kunatum Prasidthrathsint, MD[a,b,c,d,e],
Jack T. Stapleton, MD[a,c,d,e],*

KEYWORDS

- Viral hepatitis • Viral diagnostics • Hepatitis A • Hepatitis B • Hepatitis C
- Hepatitis D • Hepatitis E

KEY POINTS

- Viral hepatitis may be caused by many viruses, although 5 viruses are named for their primary manifestation of causing hepatic infection (hepatitis A, B, C, D, and E).
- Although clinical presentation of viral hepatitis is insufficient to determine cause, precise diagnosis of acute hepatitis A and B is feasible by serologic methods.
- Although definitive characterization of infection duration is not possible for hepatitis C, D, and E, diagnosis of ongoing infection is possible using serology and nucleic acid amplification methods.
- Viral hepatitis diagnostic testing is critical for treatment initiation and/or monitoring treatment response in hepatitis B, C, and D.

INTRODUCTION

The word hepatitis is derived from it is, meaning inflammation, and hepar, the Greek word for liver. Many conditions, including alcohol ingestion and medications, may cause liver inflammation. Although many viral and bacterial infections cause hepatitis (eg, cytomegalovirus, Epstein-Barr virus, influenza, yellow fever virus), 5 viruses

Disclosure: There are no relevant commercial relationships to disclose.
Funding: Department of Veterans Affairs Merit Review Grants BX000207 (J.T. Stapleton), and NIAID R56AI126493
[a] Division of Infectious Diseases, Department of Internal Medicine, University of Iowa Carver College of Medicine, Iowa City, IA, USA; [b] Division of Clinical Microbiology, Department of Pathology, University of Iowa Carver College of Medicine, Iowa City, IA, USA; [c] Department of Microbiology and Immunology, University of Iowa Carver College of Medicine, Iowa City, IA, USA; [d] University of Iowa Hospitals and Clinics, SW54, GH, 200 Hawkins Drive, Iowa City, IA 52242, USA; [e] Medicine and Research Services, Iowa City Veterans Administration Health Care Center, Iowa City, IA, USA
* Corresponding author. UIHC, SW54, GH, 200 Hawkins Drive, Iowa City, IA 52242.
E-mail address: jack-stapleton@uiowa.edu

Gastroenterol Clin N Am 48 (2019) 259–279
https://doi.org/10.1016/j.gtc.2019.02.007
0889-8553/19/Published by Elsevier Inc.

primarily infect the liver and are named after the clinical disease: hepatitis A to E. A sixth, hepatitis G virus, was initially thought to cause hepatitis, but subsequent studies did not confirm this hypothesis.[1] This virus is not discussed in this review.

Symptoms of hepatitis are not specific to a single hepatitis virus, and thus clinical presentation does not distinguish between different viral causes. Hepatitis virus infection may be mild or asymptomatic. In symptomatic cases, acute hepatitis is associated with flulike illness, fever, fatigue, loss of appetite, abdominal pain, nausea, vomiting, jaundice, dark urine, clay-colored stools, and (rarely) fulminant hepatitis. Chronic hepatitis is frequently asymptomatic or mildly symptomatic. Over time, chronic viral hepatitis may lead to persistent inflammation, leading to fibrosis with resultant cirrhosis, liver failure, and hepatocellular carcinoma.

The transmission mode for hepatitis A and E is primarily through contaminated water or food (fecal-oral), although transfusion-related hepatitis A virus (HAV) has occurred. Hepatitis B and C are transmitted through sexual and parenteral exposure, and vertically from mother to child. Hepatitis D is only transmitted with hepatitis B virus (HBV), as described later.

Microbial diagnostic testing is increasingly using molecular testing for nucleic acid testing (NAT; eg, using the polymerase chain reaction [PCR]) or microbial proteins using mass spectrometry because of their more sensitive and specific detection of pathogens. However, in viral hepatitis, serologic tests remain the mainstay of diagnosis. In some circumstances, serology requires concurrent NAT methods. Understanding hepatitis transmission modes, natural history and viral kinetics, and the limitations of testing is required for choosing appropriate diagnostic tests for viral hepatitis.

HEPATITIS A VIRUS

HAV is a positive-sense, single-strand RNA virus classified as a member of the Hepatovirus genus within the family Picornaviridae. Viral RNA is directly translated into a single polyprotein cleaved by viral proteases into structural and nonstructural protein products. Although there are 7 HAV genotypes, there is a single serotype. HAV is transmitted by ingesting contaminated food or water, and it enters the bloodstream through the oropharynx or intestinal epithelium. It is delivered to the liver, where it replicates in hepatocytes and Kupffer cells. Although classically thought of as a nonenveloped virus, recent data show that a pseudoenveloped particle is released from cells into the bloodstream or into the biliary tree. Virus released into the biliary tree is transported to the gastrointestinal tract for excretion, and the pseudoenvelope is removed from the particles by bile acids.[2] The excreted nonenveloped particles are highly resistant to environmental stress and may remain infectious for prolonged periods of time.

Most HAV infections are asymptomatic in young children; however, HAV more commonly causes disease in older children and adults. The average time from exposure to clinical illness is 4 weeks (range, 2–6 weeks), and fecal viral RNA levels rapidly decrease at the time of clinical illness (**Fig. 1**).[3] Anti-HAV antibodies and HAV-specific cytotoxic T cells are detected at the time of illness. Taken together, these findings suggest that HAV pathogenesis is immunologically mediated. Illness usually lasts less than 1 month; however, relapsing hepatitis and, rarely, fulminant hepatitis A occur. A variety of extrahepatic complications are described, including arthritis and vasculitis. Following infection, there is no residual liver disease, and anti-HAV is protective against reinfection.

Diagnostic Evaluation

HAV viremia begins before illness and virus excretion into the stool via the biliary tree peaks around the time of maximal liver enzyme level increases (see **Fig. 1**). Anti-HAV

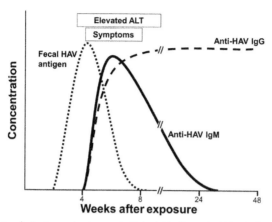

Fig. 1. The kinetics of viral, serologic, and clinical findings in HAV infection. ALT, alanine transaminase; IgM, immunoglobulin M.

antibodies are detected at or shortly after increase of alanine transaminase (ALT) level. Initially, anti-HAV immunoglobulin (Ig) M isotype antibodies are detected, and these typically decrease below detection limits within 6 months after infection. Before IgM levels decrease, anti-HAV IgG is detected. Anti-HAV IgG is protective and persists for life. Measurement of total anti-HAV antibodies identifies both IgG and IgM iso-types, and, if present, there is lifelong protection against reinfection. Total antibodies does not distinguish acute versus chronic infection. IgM-specific antibody testing is required, and, if positive, testing is diagnostic of acute infection. Because HAV is an acute self-limited disease, and IgM antibodies are present before and during infection, there is no clinical indication for detecting virus by either antigen or RNA detection methods. As a result, no commercially available HAV antigen detection or NAT assays are available.

HEPATITIS B VIRUS

HBV is an enveloped, partially double-stranded DNA virus within the family Hepadnaviridae. HBV is classified into 10 genotypes, A to J.[4] Although genotypes have distinct geographic distributions and different rates of disease progression,[4,5] clinical use of genotype determination requires further study.[6] The infectious HBV virion is composed of a lipoprotein envelope (hepatitis B surface antigen [HBsAg]), the viral hepatitis B core (HBc) protein or antigen (HBcAg), which assembles into the capsid encapsidating the partially double-stranded, circular DNA genome (**Fig. 2A**). The particle also carries the RNA-dependent DNA polymerase (RdDp or reverse transcriptase). DNA replication uses an RNA intermediate, explaining why some human immunodeficiency virus (HIV) antiviral drugs are active against HBV. The core protein precursor (precore) contains a 28-amino acid region at the N terminus. A truncated HBcAg containing the precore region is called the hepatitis B e antigen (HBeAg). This HBeAg can be secreted by infected cells and is a marker of HBV replication and infectivity.[7] HBsAg is released into the bloodstream at high concentrations in large spherical or tubular particles (**Fig. 2B, C**). Specific patterns of viral antigens and antibodies appear during acute and chronic infection. Therefore, understanding the different HBV antigens is critical for interpreting diagnostic tests for HBV infection.

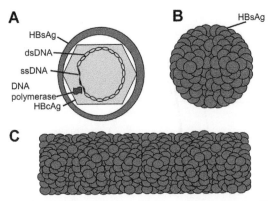

Fig. 2. HBV virus particles. (*A*) The infectious (Dane) particle contains HBsAg, the partially double-stranded DNA (dsDNA) genome, the viral RNA-dependent DNA polymerase, and HBcAg. HBsAg is released into serum as spherical particles (*B*) or tubular structures (*C*). These particles do not carry viral DNA, HBcAg, or the viral polymerase. ssDNA, single-strand DNA.

Natural History

HBV primarily infects hepatocytes, although viral DNA is also detected in peripheral blood mononuclear cells. Viral DNA is detected in serum using NAT methods within 2 to 5 days after acquisition.[8,9] DNA detection is highly sensitive and thus a reliable marker of active HBV replication. HBsAg is detected using serologic methods and is detected 1 to 2 weeks after HBV DNA detection.[10] HBsAg detection indicates active HBV replication. Because viral replication can be determined serologically, HBV DNA is usually not tested until HBsAg is detected.

Less than 15% of patients with HBV infection have clinical hepatitis, and less than half of these developed jaundice.[11] Clinical illness correlates with the age and immunologic maturity, and newborns and children rarely have significant clinical disease. Overall, approximately 95% of immunocompetent people infected with HBV have self-limited HBV infection, most recovering completely. The remaining individuals develop chronic infection. The rate of viremia clearance is inversely related to the magnitude of clinical illness; thus chronic infection is increased in newborns and immune compromised individuals who rarely have overt hepatitis.[11,12] Vertical transmission from mothers infected with HBV to their children results in chronic infection in approximately 90% of cases.[13]

Symptomatic patients may have a preicteric or prodromal period followed by clinical hepatitis that typically occurs 11 to 24 weeks following exposure.[8,9] Peak liver enzyme level increases occur after development of HBV-specific immune responses, supporting an immune-mediated component of HBV liver pathogenesis. In those with clinical illness, symptoms generally improve by the time jaundice develops, typically 2 to 6 weeks after peak serum HBV DNA levels. In acute, self-limited infection, HBV DNA and HBsAg levels generally decrease below detection limits in the first 3 to 4 months after infection.[8]

Serologic evaluation of infection

Hepatitis B virus core antigen and antibody The first antibodies to appear are directed against the core protein (anti-HBc; **Fig. 3**). The first anti-HBc antibodies are IgM isotype, and these switch to the IgG isotype over 3 to 6 months. Once anti-HBc IgG antibodies develop, they are detected for life in most individuals, and measurement of

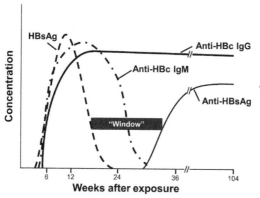

Fig. 3. Viral and serologic findings in acute HBV infection. "Window" is time between positive surface antigen and antibody, which is not detected unless anti-HBc antibodies are measured.

total anti-HBc (detecting IgG and IgM anti-HBc isotypes) is the best marker for documenting prior HBV infection regardless of other serologic results. Total anti-HBc does not indicate the timing of infection, and anti-HBc IgM measurement is needed to determine whether the infection is recent (see **Fig. 3; Fig. 4**).

Hepatitis B virus surface antigen and antibody In acute self-limited infection, antibodies to HBsAg are detected after HBsAg clearance and appearance of anti-HBc IgG. Anti–hepatitis B surface antigen (HBs) is generally detected within 6 months after infection and is a marker of protection against reinfection.[14] Current HBV vaccines are composed of recombinant (noninfectious) HBsAg particles that elicit anti-HBs (see **Fig. 2B, C**), thus vaccinated individuals have anti-HBs antibodies detected in serum.[14] The presence or absence of total anti-HBc differentiates prior infection from vaccination in hepatitis B surface antibody (HBsAb)–positive people, because vaccination does not elicit anti-HBc.[13] Because there is a period of time (window) when HBsAg and anti-HBs are both negative during acute infection, screening for HBV infection should include a total anti-HBc test (see **Fig. 3**).

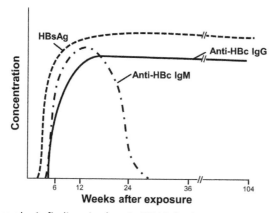

Fig. 4. Viral and serologic findings in chronic HBV infection.

Although the patterns in **Figs. 3** and **4** are highly consistent, one serologic pattern occurs that is difficult to reconcile with clinical decision making. Specifically, HBV DNA without detectable anti-HBc occurs in immunocompromised people with acute hepatitis (13.8%), in HBV reactivation (41.4%), and chronic hepatitis B (44.8%).[15–18] Approximately half of these patients develop anti-HBc over time (often at low levels), or HBc is detected using different anti-HBc assays.[18] No mutations have been identified in core protein sequences in these individuals, thus this scenario seems to represent an immune recognition defect.[18] Therefore, it is not advisable to rely on a single anti-HBc–negative result to exclude HBV infection in immunocompromised hosts and repeat anti-HBc testing or using different serologic testing methods should be considered.[18]

Hepatitis B virus e antigen and antibody HBeAg is a variant of the HBcAg and is released into the circulation shortly after infection. Development of anti-HBe and loss of HBeAg during acute self-limited infection is a predictor of clearance. In chronic infection, development of anti-HBe occurs late in infection, usually after several years. Seroconversion to anti-HBe indicates a favorable outcome marking transition from high replication rates to low replication rates associated with inactive hepatitis B. However, some individuals with anti-HBe show active liver disorder. Mutations in the precore amino acid sequence have been identified, suggesting that mutation resulted in seroconversion to anti-HBe.[19,20]

Chronic hepatitis B virus infection
Chronic HBV infection is defined as detection of HBsAg on at least 2 separate occasions measured at least 6 months apart.[21,22] Host cellular immune responses to virus-infected hepatocytes are thought to be responsible for hepatic inflammation causing liver injury. These responses contribute to the development of cirrhosis and hepatocellular carcinoma in chronic HBV infection. There are 4 phases in chronic HBV that are important in deciding when to treat HBV. These are summarized as follows:

1. Immunotolerance. Asymptomatic patients with positive HBsAg, HBeAg, and normal liver enzyme levels. High HBV DNA (>20,000 international units [IU]/mL).
2. HBeAg-positive immunoactive disease. Individual may or may not have clinical liver disease. Positive HBsAg and HBeAg, positive or negative anti-HBe, increased liver enzyme levels (>2 times the upper limit of normal ALT level), and high HBV DNA (>20,000 IU/mL).
3. HBeAg-negative, inactive disease (inactive chronic HBV or low replicative infection). Positive HBsAg, negative HBeAg (positive anti-HBe), normal ALT level, low HBV DNA level (<2000 IU/mL). There may be fibrosis from previous inflammation.
4. HBeAg-negative immunoreactive disease. Negative HBsAg, HBeAg (positive anti-HBe), increased liver enzyme levels (>2 times upper limits of normal ALT), intermediate to high HBV DNA level (>2000 IU/mL).

Although these phases of HBV pathogenesis do not have unique clinical presentations, disease is generally asymptomatic in the immunotolerance and HBeAg-negative inactive disease phase but more active in the HBeAg-positive immunoactive and HBeAg-negative immunoreactive disease stages. Because either HBeAg-positive immunoactive disease or HBeAg-negative immunoreactivation disease may progress to liver failure, initiation of treatment is recommended in these situations. HBV DNA levels may fluctuate, although they are persistently increased (>20,000 IU/mL) in individuals with detectable HBeAg. HBV DNA can differentiate inactive carriers from patients with HBeAg-negative chronic hepatitis B.[23] Patients with inactive chronic hepatitis B typically have HBV DNA levels less than 2000 IU/mL, whereas those with immune active hepatitis B have HBV DNA levels greater than 20,000 IU/mL.

DIAGNOSTIC TESTING
Virus Detection

Hepatitis B surface antigen and hepatitis B e antigen detection

HBV antigens are detected using solid-phase immunoassays. HBsAg particles or HBeAg protein is captured to the solid phase with monoclonal or polyclonal sera and a labeled secondary antibody to the specific antigen is used for detection. These assays use microparticles and are automated. Current detection methods use enzymatic, chemiluminescence, or fluorescence polarization methods to detect the antigens.[24] HBsAg assays detect a minimum of 0.7 ng/mL of HBsAg, with newer tests having detection limits down to 0.13 ng/mL.[25]

There are concerns that some assays cannot detect HBsAg variants with mutations in the major antigenic region that result in conformation changes. Many HBsAg immunoassays use antibodies directed against the main antigenic (a) determinant. Mutation in this region may account for the false-negative results by some assays.[26–28] Thus, acute infection should always include screening for anti-HBc or HBV DNA.[29] HBsAg quantitation is not needed in patients with chronic hepatitis B, although quantitative HBsAg has been used in monitoring patients receiving interferon-based therapies.[22]

Nucleic acid amplification testing

Hepatitis B virus DNA polymerase chain reaction Quantitative HBV DNA testing is essential for determining the need for HBV treatment and for evaluating treatment response.[22] Highly sensitivity NAT assays are important for diagnosis of HBeAg-negative chronic HBV and occult HBV, in which DNA concentration may be low.[30] Current HBV DNA quantification methods use real-time PCR, which has excellent analytical performance, including a low limit of detection and a broad linear range.[30] However, characteristics vary among different commercial platforms. The World Health Organization (WHO) has generated an HBV DNA standard and results should be provided in IU.[31] Nevertheless, quantitative results may vary and the best practice for following DNA levels is to use the same assay from the same laboratory whenever possible.[30]

Serology

Anti–hepatitis B core, anti–hepatitis B surface, and anti–hepatitis B e

Commercial detection of anti-HBc, anti-HBs, and anti-HBe antibodies uses enzyme-linked immunosorbent assay (ELISA) methodologies. Several versions of each test are available using different detection methods and instrumentation. The 2 most commonly used methods use a competitive approach (anti-HBc and anti-HBe) or a solid-phase, sandwich-type approach (anti-HBs).[14,32]

Genotype Testing

At present, commercial testing of HBV genotypes is not recommended for clinical care, with the exception of testing before interferon-based therapy or when knowledge of the HBV genotype may aid risk stratification of disease progression.[21,22]

Resistance Testing

Because transmission of resistance mutations is rare in North America, resistance testing is not recommended in treatment-naive patients before starting therapy.[33] Antiviral resistance may be useful for patients with past treatment experience, those with persistent or virological breakthrough while on antiviral therapy as defined by a 10-fold increase in serum HBV DNA from their nadir during treatment.[22] Resistance is determined by evaluating specific sequence variation within the polymerase gene and identifying polymorphisms known to correlate with antiviral resistance in vitro or in vivo. Current methods include restriction fragment length polymorphism, hybridization, and sequencing methodologies, and testing usually requires HBV DNA concentrations greater than 1000 IU/mL.

LABORATORY USE IN MONITORING
Baseline Studies

Patients with chronic HBV infection should be evaluated to determine the phase of infection as described earlier. ALT, HBV DNA, and HBeAg should be measured, and liver fibrosis quantified to allow prediction of long-term outcomes and inform treatment decisions. In patients receiving treatment, HBV DNA levels are the primary method to determine treatment response. Therefore, serial testing of hepatic function, quantitative HBV DNA, HBeAg, anti-HBe, as well as evaluation of liver fibrosis are needed to guide treatment decisions.[21,22] In addition to HBV testing, laboratory monitoring during antiviral therapy should include measurement of HBsAg, HBeAg, anti-HBs, anti-HBe, and complete blood count (CBC), and renal and hepatic function every 3 to 6 months. These tests potentially identify progression of liver disease, extrahepatic manifestations of chronic HBV, and treatment toxicities.[21] A summary of serologic and NAT results useful in different HBV clinical situations is shown in **Table 1**.

HEPATITIS C VIRUS

Hepatitis C Virus (HCV) is a positive-sense, single-stranded RNA virus. Its structure, genomic organization, and replication cycle support classification as a member of the family Flaviviridae, but are unique enough to classify it in a separate genus, Hepacivirus.[1] The RNA genome is translated into a polyprotein that is cleaved by cellular and viral proteases into structural and nonstructural proteins. Because of extensive genetic diversity, there are 7 major genotypes and 67 HCV subtypes globally.[34] Genotype distribution varies by geographic location,[34] and, globally, genotype 1 is the predominant genotype, followed by genotype 3, then genotype 4.[35]

Natural History

Acute HCV refers to the first 6 months following acquisition of infection, regardless of symptoms.[36,37] Infection is usually asymptomatic despite abnormal liver function test results.[38,39] In symptomatic patients, most present with nonspecific flulike symptoms.[36] A minority of infected individuals develop symptoms of acute viral hepatitis, including jaundice, anorexia, and abdominal discomfort.[36] Although HCV infection

| Table 1 | | | | | |
| Diagnostic test patterns in acute and chronic hepatitis B virus infection | | | | | |
HBsAg	Anti-HBs	Anti-HBc IgM	Total Anti-HBc	HBV DNA	Interpretation
+	−	+	+/−	+	Acute hepatitis B
−	+	−	+	−	Past infection
−	+	−	−	−	Vaccination
−	−	−	+	+/−	Previous infection, occult hepatitis B

may cause lifelong infection, 15% to 30% of infections resolve spontaneously.[40,41] These patients lose detectable HCV RNA, and, in symptomatic patients, this typically occurs within 3 to 4 months following the onset of symptoms.[42] Several variables are associated with HCV clearance, including polymorphisms in the interferon-lambda-2 gene (IL28B), sex, race, age, and a variety of host immune markers (human leukocyte antigen [HLA]-B, HLA-C, Killer-cell immunoglobulin-like receptor (KIR)).[43,44] The timing of viral clearance influences the decision to consider therapy for acute hepatitis.[45]

However, most patients have persistent viremia. Chronic HCV infection is defined as lasting more than 6 months. Chronic infection is usually asymptomatic and may progress slowly and silently to chronic liver disease.[41] The major liver disease caused by HCV is fibrosis, and severe fibrosis (cirrhosis) develops in 20% to 30% of chronic HCV infections.[41] Although cirrhosis can develop rapidly, it typically develops over 20 to 30 years. Several factors increase the risk of cirrhosis, including alcohol use, male sex, age of acquisition, and immune suppression (HIV).[41,46] People infected with HCV with cirrhosis are also at increased risk of hepatocellular carcinoma. Several extrahepatic manifestations of HCV are also recognized, including arthritis, keratoconjunctivitis sicca, lichen planus, glomerulonephritis, porphyria cutanea tarda, and type II cryoglobulinemia.[41] Up to 80% of people infected with HCV have detectable rheumatoid factor in serum; half of these also have cryoglobulins detected.[47]

Hepatitis C Virus Kinetics

HCV RNA is not detected in serum during the first 1 to 2 weeks following transmission,[48] but HCV RNA is the earliest marker of infection.[38] Early in infection, HCV RNA levels range widely (from 2500 to >1 million IU/mL). Viremia precedes ALT and bilirubin increases. The HCV RNA pattern early in infection often shows a peak, followed by a reduction in concentration. In patients who spontaneously clear infection, HCV RNA continues to rapidly decrease until viremia is not detectable.[49,50] An alternative pattern is sometimes seen, in which low-level viremia (<120 copies/mL) may precede an increase and plateau of HCV viral load (VL).[38,51] The variability emphasizes the need to repeat HCV RNA testing in situations in which the suspicion of early HCV is high. Most people with chronic HCV infection have fluctuating or high HCV RNA levels.[40,50] HCV RNA levels frequently stabilize somewhat, and, although there is a large range of concentrations between individuals, average HCV RNA levels are more than 1 million genome copies per milliliter of plasma.[52]

Seroconversion is generally slow, ranging from 34 to 70 days in HIV-negative blood product recipients and intravenous drug users.[53,54] Antibodies are rarely detected before liver enzyme levels peak or return to normal values. Thus, infection may be missed if liver enzyme levels alone are used as the indication for HCV testing.[38] The delay is even greater in individuals infected with HIV, with median seroconversion ranging from 91 to 158 days.[55] Antibody-negative, HCV RNA–positive infection is uncommon but occurs in individuals both infected and uninfected with HIV.[56,57] Although the reasons for variation in viremia and host immune response patterns are not clear, they likely are influenced by several factors, including the route of entry, the nature of inoculum, the frequency of exposure, and viral-mediated interference with host immune responses.[58,59]

Diagnostic Testing

Diagnostic testing for HCV infection relies primarily on the detection of antibodies by serologic testing and the direct detection of viral RNA by NAT. Both HCV serology and NAT are validated and US Food and Drug Administration (FDA) approved, using serum or plasma as the specimen source. There is also a licensed serologic assay performed using oral fluid.[60]

Detection of virus

Antigen detection Detection and quantification of core antigen in serum or plasma uses ELISA. This assay is used extensively in Europe and is available globally, particularly in resource-limited settings because of target stability, simple instrumentation, and cost.[50] Detection of HCV core antigen usually correlates well with HCV RNA detection and thus may serve as a surrogate marker for viral replication.[61,62] However, the assay has inferior sensitivity and specificity compared with HCV RNA testing when HCV RNA values are less than 20,000 IU/mL. Therefore, this method is not commonly used in the United States.[61,62]

Nucleic acid detection testing HCV can be quantified using target amplification techniques (transcription-mediated amplification [TMA], or reverse transcription real-time PCR) methods with very low limits of detection, ranging from 1.0 to 1.7 $\log_{10}$ IU/mL. Quantitative methods are preferred to qualitative methods for establishing baseline HCV RNA concentration before treatment and for following response during and following therapy. The American Association for the Study of Liver Diseases (AASLD) recommends use of FDA-approved, highly sensitive HCV VL with a limit of detection of less than 25 IU/mL.[63]

In the past, quantitative units of various assays did not report the same concentration of HCV RNA in clinical samples. The WHO established an international calibration standard for HCV RNA and defined it as IU per milliliter to allow comparison of HCV RNA levels in clinical samples between laboratories and assays. Nevertheless, some problems remain because of intrinsic variability between instruments and laboratories, including precision, reproducibility, and accuracy.[64] It is important to remember that, because the methods rely on logarithmic amplification of viral RNA, VL changes less than 0.5 $\log_{10}$ IU/mL (eg, 3-fold) may reflect differences in laboratory performance.[65]

Serology

Available HCV serologic assays in the United States include the second-generation and third-generation enzyme immunoassay (EIA). No single HCV antigen consistently elicits antibodies in humans, thus the assays use multiple HCV antigens. The first-generation HCV assay used a region of the nonstructural protein NS4 (c100-3) to detect anti-HCV antibodies (**Fig. 5**). This assay was refined in second-generation tests to use regions of NS4 (regions termed C200, HC-31), NS3 (protease; c33c), and core (c22-3) proteins. This assay was further enhanced in third-generation tests and the core antigen and NS4 antigens were changed (c22p, a peptide containing a major epitope residing in the core protein between amino acids 10–35), NS4 HC-31 to NS4 5-1-1p, and the NS5 protein was added. Second-generation and third-generation EIA tests have increased sensitivity and specificity and identify early seroconversion and atypical seroconversion better than first-generation tests.[66]

Although second-generation assays are still available, they may yield false-negative results, and alternative testing with third-generation EIA or NAT should be considered in patients with negative EIA 2.0 results, particularly in those with a high index of suspicion.

In addition to the standard EIA tests, there is an FDA-approved, rapid, highly accurate point-of-care test available. It detects antibody using an indirect immunoassay technique using a nitrocellulose membrane coated with core, NS3, and NS4

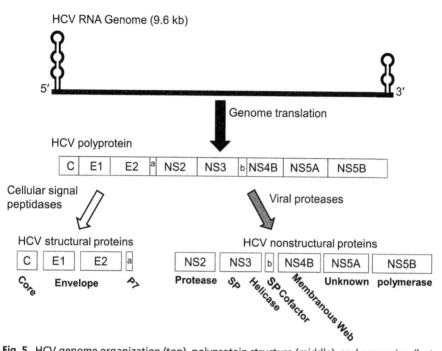

Fig. 5. HCV genome organization (top), polyprotein structure (middle), and processing (bottom). The 5′ and 3′ untranslated regions contain highly structured, stem-loop regions. [a] P7; [b] NS4A; SP, serine protease.

antigens. The clinical performance is comparable with current laboratory-developed EIA methods, and this test may prove useful in addressing the problem of underdiagnosis of HCV.[60] IgM testing has no utility in acute hepatitis C because it may be detected at the same time as IgG and may persist for up to a year after HCV acquisition.[67]

Genotype and resistance testing

As noted earlier, there are 7 HCV genotypes. Determining the HCV genotype is useful for determining the best treatment regimen, particularly in the era of interferon (IFN)-based treatments. In addition, many direct-acting antiviral (DAA) anti-HCV therapies are genotype or subtype specific.[68] HCV genotypes are determined using Sanger sequencing, next-generation sequencing (deep sequencing), or hybridization methods, and can use short regions of the 5′ untranslated genome sequence from samples and align these with reference sequences.[69]

Because of the error-prone HCV RNA-dependent RNA polymerase, HCV amino acid polymorphisms naturally occur throughout the genome coding region that may be associated with resistance or reduced susceptibility to a member or even an entire class of DAAs. These sequence differences may or may not confer resistance to a specific drug in the class (eg, protease inhibitor, polymerase inhibitor, NS5A inhibitor). In addition, resistance mutations may be selected during DAA treatment. DAA HCV therapy is rapidly evolving, and there are increasing options for pangenotypic inhibitors. Thus, the use of genotype and resistance testing is constantly changing. The AASLD provides and updates recommendation guidelines.[63]

DIAGNOSTIC APPROACH FOR HEPATITIS C

At present, there are no validated methods to distinguish acute and chronic HCV infection.[70] Infection duration estimation relies on prior diagnostic testing results and an understanding of the mode of transmission, natural history, viral kinetics, and limitations of different laboratory test methodologies. Because seroconversion may be delayed for many weeks following exposure, diagnosis of HCV during acute infection requires HCV RNA detection.[45] Further, HCV RNA may be negative or very low titer early in infection, thus repeat RNA testing is warranted 2 to 4 weeks following a negative test in cases in which there is a high index of suspicion.[50]

Detection of HCV RNA without anti-HCV strongly indicates acute hepatitis in immunocompetent patients, particularly when it is followed by seroconversion.[50] In clinical practice, this sequence of events is uncommonly detected. Most individuals with chronic HCV infection have positive RNA and antibody results, although infection occasionally does not seem to elicit detectable antibodies.[50] Therefore, diagnosis in these patients should rely on HCV RNA. **Table 2** provides a summary of diagnostic tests and interpretations.

LABORATORY MONITORING

Monitoring should follow AASLD guidelines (www.HCVGuidance.org on March 19, 2018).[63]

Baseline Laboratories

The HCV genotype should be determined in patients with chronic HCV infection, because it contributes to treatment options and prognosis. Resistance testing is also needed in some situations. At present it is recommended for some anti-NS5A DAA therapies as a baseline in genotypes 1a and 3. However, this is an evolving field, and consultation with AASLD guidelines is highly recommended before treating HCV infection.[63] Other laboratory studies needed before initiating HCV DAA therapy include CBC, electrolytes, renal function, liver enzymes, PT/INR, serologic evaluation for HIV and HBV, and an assessment of hepatic fibrosis. Methods to assess fibrosis include liver biopsy, imaging, and noninvasive markers (ie, fibroscan).[71]

Table 2
Summary of laboratory result and interpretation

Anti-HCV Ab	HCV RNA	Interpretation
Negative	Detectable	• Acute hepatitis C • Chronic hepatitis C in immunocompromised or exceptional cases
Detected	Undetectable	• Spontaneous resolved[a] • Treated infection
Detected	Detected	• Chronic infection • Acute infection (clinical history of exposure may help to distinguish)
Negative	Undetectable	• No evidence of hepatitis C infection[b]

Abbreviation: Ab, antibody.
[a] May require repeat HCV RNA testing to ensure the clearance.
[b] May require repeat HCV RNA testing if high clinical suspicion of early infection within 1 to 2 weeks of acquisition is suspected.

During therapy, CBC, creatinine level, and liver enzyme levels are recommended 4 weeks after starting treatment and as clinically indicated for drug-related adverse effects. Quantitative HCV RNA testing is recommended 4 weeks after starting and 12 weeks after completing therapy. Testing may be considered at the end of treatment and 24 weeks or longer following the completion of therapy.[63]

HEPATITIS D VIRUS

Hepatitis D virus (HDV) is a defective RNA virus. Because HDV requires the HBV lipid envelope (HBsAg; see **Fig. 2**) to assemble into viral particles that are capable of infecting new cells, it is incapable of reproducing unless there is HBV coinfection.[72] HDV is a member of the Deltavirus genus and there are 8 genotypes (genotypes 1–8), which have distinct and specific geographic distributions.[73]

HDV can be cotransmitted with HBV to people who do not have HBV infection (**Fig. 6**). Alternatively, HDV may superinfect individuals with existing HBV infection (**Fig. 7**).[74] Clinically, infection with HDV is indistinguishable from the other viral hepatitis viruses, although on average hepatitis is more severe.[75] In acute coinfection, HDV clears if HBV clears, thus approximately 95% of these infections resolve. HDV seems to be more aggressive, leading to more rapid cirrhosis and hepatocellular disease in individuals chronically infected with HBV and superinfected with HDV.[76] HDV becomes chronic in 70% to 90% of superinfections.[75] HDV transmission risks are the same as HBV, although infections are highest in injecting drug users; people exposed to blood or blood products; and individuals from Mediterranean, sub-Sahara Africa, the Middle East, the northern part of South America, and central and northern Asia.[77] Guidelines recommend screening for HDV in immigrants from regions with high HDV endemicity, individuals infected with HBV with unexplained high ALT levels, and in those with uncertainty regarding HBV treatment initiation.[22]

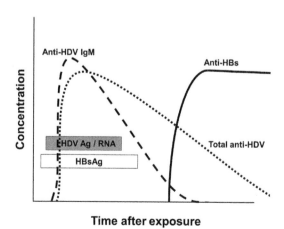

Time after exposure

Fig. 6. The kinetics of viral and serologic findings in HDV coinfection with HBV in a self-limited HBV infection. Because HBsAg serves as the surface envelope protein for HDV, it must be present when HDV RNA is detected. HBV serology as in **Fig. 3**. HDV Ag, hepatitis delta virus antigen.

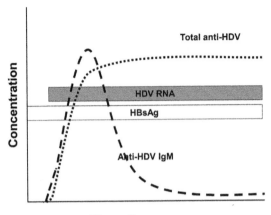

Fig. 7. The kinetics of viral and serologic findings in HDV superinfection of a person with chronic HBV infection. Because HBsAg serves as the surface envelope protein for HDV, it must be present when HDV RNA is detected. HBV serology as in **Fig. 4**.

Diagnostic Testing

Virus detection

Hepatitis D virus antigen Detection of HDV antigen (HDAg) is an indicator of acute infection.[78] It appears early, but is very short lived. Serum HDAg can be detected by either ELISA or radioimmunoassay, but is less sensitive than measuring HDV RNA.

Hepatitis D virus RNA Quantitative HDV RNA represents the gold standard for diagnosis of HDV infection and is useful for monitoring response to treatment, especially to assess a sustained virologic response, which is associated with cure.[79,80] Available assays may not detect HDV RNA and, if they do, the measured RNA levels may be dramatically lower than actual levels, especially when measuring the African HDV genotypes (HDV-5 to HDV-8). This finding is attributed to sequence diversity causing primer mismatches, and potentially to the complex secondary structure of genomic RNA.[81] New instruments are under development to improve performance characteristics regardless of the genotype.[82] The WHO has developed an international standard HDV RNA preparation (WHO-HDV-IS) to serve as a quality control.[83] Further, a commercially available automated quantitative real-time PCR method is available in reference laboratories in the United States.

Anti–Hepatitis D virus antibodies Serologic testing for HDV infection uses anti-HDV IgM antibody detection. Anti-HDV IgM is detected during the window period between HDAg and development of anti-HDV IgG (see **Fig. 6**). Anti-HDV IgM indicates chronic infection when present at high titer.[78] It rapidly declines in patients with self-limited infection. In contrast, anti-HDV IgM persists in patients with chronic infection.[84,85] Decreasing anti-HDV IgM level predicts resolution of chronic HDV infection, which may occur spontaneously or be induced by anti-HBV therapy. Anti-HDV IgM increases in response to HDV-induced liver damage[86] and may be useful if HDV RNA is negative when there are clinical features suggesting HDV-related liver disease, given the poor sensitivity of HDV RNA assays.[87] Anti-HDV IgG appears several weeks after anti-HDV IgM and may persist for life regardless of clinical outcome or clearance of infection.[85]

The AASLD recommends screening by measuring anti-HDV antibodies (IgM and IgG). If either of these is positive, HDV RNA testing is indicated to diagnose active infection.[22]

Laboratory Use in Monitoring

Baseline laboratories

Evaluation for treatment follows the same approach used for HBV, and includes liver enzymes, HBV DNA, and fibrosis evaluation.[22] Anti-HBc IgM can be used to determine the status of acute coinfection (anti-HBc IgM positive) versus HDV infection of a chronic HBV carrier (anti-HBc IgM negative). This approach provides some insight into the potential of developing chronic HDV infection.

There are no HDV-specific antiviral therapies, but treating HBV effectively treats HDV. IFN-based therapies may have HDV effects. Monitoring HDV RNA during HBV therapy provides no predictive benefit. If an IFN-based therapy is used, HDV RNA should be monitored up to 24 weeks after completing treatment to determine whether HDV clears regardless of HBV. However, although IFN is the drug of choice for HDV, treatment success rates are less than 60%.[22,79,88]

HEPATITIS E VIRUS

Hepatitis E virus (HEV) is a nonenveloped RNA virus classified within the Hepeviridae family. There are at least 4 genotypes; genotypes 1 and 2 are found exclusively in humans, whereas genotypes 3 and 4 are zoonoses found in humans and other animals. There are at least 2 distinct epidemiologic patterns. HEV1 and HEV2 are associated with large sporadic and epidemic outbreaks in developing countries. HEV is transmitted by the fecal-oral route, usually via contaminated water. Autochthonous cases of sporadic hepatitis in the developed world are associated with HEV3 and HEV4 infection, which are thought to be transmitted zoonotically by ingesting under-cooked animal products (swine, deer, and unidentified sources) in addition to travelers visiting endemic regions.[89-91] HEV should be considered in cases of unexplained acute hepatitis regardless of travel history.[91] Although it was thought that HEV only caused acute, self-limited infection, it seems that HEV may cause chronic hepatitis resulting in rapidly progressing cirrhosis in immunocompromised hosts, including patients receiving kidney transplants and those with HIV-1 infection.[92-94]

Diagnostic Testing

Although there are no FDA-approved tests at present, many commercial and reference laboratories have quantitative HEV RNA and serology for HEV available.

Detection of virus

Hepatitis E virus RNA HEV RNA is detected using NAT methodologies, although no serologic method is available for HEV antigen. In patients with acute HEV infection, viremia peaks during the incubation period and early symptomatic phase (**Fig. 8**).[95,96] HEV fecal excretion is short lived and HEV RNA is not generally detected in serum or feces following biochemical hepatitis.[95] In immunocompromised patients in whom HEV RNA persists for 3 months or longer, it seems unlikely that spontaneous viral clearance will occur.[97] Recently, the WHO developed an international standard RNA preparation for genotype 3a to facilitate accurate quantification of HEV RNA between laboratories.

Diagnostic testing

Anti-HEV IgM level generally peaks before clinical illness, although levels remain high for approximately 8 weeks before rapidly decreasing. In general, anti-HEV IgM levels are below the level of detection by 32 weeks after illness.[96] However, the sensitivity of the assay is highly variable for different genotypes, and validated assays having the best performance characteristics are recommended.[98]

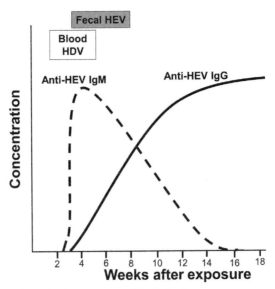

Fig. 8. Viral and serologic findings in acute HEV infection.

Anti-HEV IgG is often present in patients at the time of acute hepatitis. Anti-HEV IgG levels peak approximately 4 weeks after symptom onset and remain at high levels for more than a year.[96]

Diagnosis of acute HEV is based on the detection of anti-HEV IgM and HEV RNA.[96] Screening uses total and IgM-specific anti-HEV. If positive, HEV RNA levels should be measured. For individuals with HEV RNA detected, repeat testing is recommended. Chronic HEV infection is defined as having HEV RNA detected for a minimum of 3 months.[97]

Exceptions to the rule Chronic infection with HEV is rare, but several reports describe persistent genotype 3 HEV viremia in immunocompromised hosts with rapidly progressive liver disease.[93,94] Further confirmation of these reports in different geographic regions will be important for understanding the impact of this entity. Chronic HEV viremia without active hepatitis has been seen in individuals with HIV infection.[92] Because anti-HEV IgM and/or IgG may not be elicited in patients with severe immunosuppression, the diagnosis of HEV may be challenging.[99] Therefore, in immunocompromised patients, a combination of IgM and IgG serology and NAT detection of viral RNA should be performed. Additional testing through an independent secondary source, such as the US Centers for Disease Control and Prevention, which offers ELISA for HEV antibody as well as fecal and serum HEV NAT, should also be considered.[100]

REFERENCES

1. Stapleton JT, Foung S, Muerhoff AS, et al. The GB viruses: a review and proposed classification of GBV-A, GBV-C (HGV), and GBV-D in genus Pegivirus within the family Flaviviridae. J Gen Virol 2011;92(Pt 2):233–46.
2. Hirai-Yuki A, Hensley L, Whitmire JK, et al. Biliary secretion of quasi-enveloped human hepatitis A virus. mBio 2016;7(6) [pii:e01998-16].

3. Brown EA, Stapleton JT. Hepatitis A. In: Murray PR, Baron EJ, Jorgensen JH, et al, editors. Manual of clinical microbiology. 8th edition. Washington, DC: ASM Press; 2003. p. 1452–63.

4. Sunbul M. Hepatitis B virus genotypes: global distribution and clinical importance. World J Gastroenterol 2014;20(18):5427–34.

5. Chotiyaputta W, Lok AS. Hepatitis B virus variants. Nat Rev Gastroenterol Hepatol 2009;6(8):453–62.

6. Liang TJ. Hepatitis B: the virus and disease. Hepatology 2009;49(5 Suppl): S13–21.

7. Liang TJ, Ghany M. Hepatitis B e antigen–the dangerous endgame of hepatitis B. N Engl J Med 2002;347(3):208–10.

8. Whalley SA, Murray JM, Brown D, et al. Kinetics of acute hepatitis B virus infection in humans. J Exp Med 2001;193(7):847–54.

9. Pawlotsky JM. Hepatitis B virus (HBV) DNA assays (methods and practical use) and viral kinetics. J Hepatol 2003;39(Suppl 1):S31–5.

10. Zaaijer HL, Vrielink H, Koot M. Early detection of hepatitis B surface antigen and detection of HBsAg mutants: a comparison of five assays. Vox Sang 2001;81(4): 219–21.

11. McMahon BJ, Alward WL, Hall DB, et al. Acute hepatitis B virus infection: relation of age to the clinical expression of disease and subsequent development of the carrier state. J Infect Dis 1985;151(4):599–603.

12. Pol S. Management of HBV in immunocompromised patients. Liver Int 2013; 33(Suppl 1):182–7.

13. Bauer T, Sprinzl M, Protzer U. Immune control of hepatitis B virus. Dig Dis 2011; 29(4):423–33.

14. Cavalieri SJ, Hrabovsky S, Jorgensen T. Comparison of DiaSorin and Bio-Rad test kits for the detection of hepatitis B virus total core and surface antibodies on the Bio-Rad Evolis. Am J Clin Pathol 2010;133(1):110–3.

15. Awerkiew S, Daumer M, Reiser M, et al. Reactivation of an occult hepatitis B virus escape mutant in an anti-HBs positive, anti-HBc negative lymphoma patient. J Clin Virol 2007;38(1):83–6.

16. Avettand-Fenoel V, Thabut D, Katlama C, et al. Immune suppression as the etiology of failure to detect anti-HBc antibodies in patients with chronic hepatitis B virus infection. J Clin Microbiol 2006;44(6):2250–3.

17. Feeney SA, McCaughey C, Watt AP, et al. Reactivation of occult hepatitis B virus infection following cytotoxic lymphoma therapy in an anti-HBc negative patient. J Med Virol 2013;85(4):597–601.

18. Anastasiou OE, Widera M, Verheyen J, et al. Clinical course and core variability in HBV infected patients without detectable anti-HBc antibodies. J Clin Virol 2017;93:46–52.

19. Grandjacques C, Pradat P, Stuyver L, et al. Rapid detection of genotypes and mutations in the pre-core promoter and the pre-core region of hepatitis B virus genome: correlation with viral persistence and disease severity. J Hepatol 2000; 33(3):430–9.

20. Brunetto MR, Giarin MM, Oliveri F, et al. Wild-type and e antigen-minus hepatitis B viruses and course of chronic hepatitis. Proc Natl Acad Sci U S A 1991;88(10): 4186–90.

21. Tang LSY, Covert E, Wilson E, et al. Chronic hepatitis B infection: a review. JAMA 2018;319(17):1802–13.

22. Terrault NA, Lok ASF, McMahon BJ, et al. Update on prevention, diagnosis, and treatment of chronic hepatitis B: AASLD 2018 hepatitis B guidance. Hepatology 2018;67(4):1560–99.

23. Chu CJ, Hussain M, Lok AS. Quantitative serum HBV DNA levels during different stages of chronic hepatitis B infection. Hepatology 2002;36(6):1408–15.

24. Weber B, Bayer A, Kirch P, et al. Improved detection of hepatitis B virus surface antigen by a new rapid automated assay. J Clin Microbiol 1999;37(8):2639–47.

25. Biswas R, Tabor E, Hsia CC, et al. Comparative sensitivity of HBV NATs and HBsAg assays for detection of acute HBV infection. Transfusion 2003;43(6):788–98.

26. Jongerius JM, Wester M, Cuypers HT, et al. New hepatitis B virus mutant form in a blood donor that is undetectable in several hepatitis B surface antigen screening assays. Transfusion 1998;38(1):56–9.

27. Louisirirotchanakul S, Kanoksinsombat C, Theamboonlert A, et al. Mutation of the "a" determinant of HBsAg with discordant HBsAg diagnostic kits. Viral Immunol 2004;17(3):440–4.

28. Gerlich WH, Bremer C, Saniewski M, et al. Occult hepatitis B virus infection: detection and significance. Dig Dis 2010;28(1):116–25.

29. Allain JP, Mihaljevic I, Gonzalez-Fraile MI, et al. Infectivity of blood products from donors with occult hepatitis B virus infection. Transfusion 2013;53(7):1405–15.

30. Valsamakis A. Molecular testing in the diagnosis and management of chronic hepatitis B. Clin Microbiol Rev 2007;20(3):426–39, table of contents.

31. Saldanha J, Gerlich W, Lelie N, et al. An international collaborative study to establish a World Health Organization international standard for hepatitis B virus DNA nucleic acid amplification techniques. Vox Sang 2001;80(1):63–71.

32. Huzly D, Schenk T, Jilg W, et al. Comparison of nine commercially available assays for quantification of antibody response to hepatitis B virus surface antigen. J Clin Microbiol 2008;46(4):1298–306.

33. Lok AS, Ganova-Raeva L, Cloonan Y, et al. Prevalence of hepatitis B antiviral drug resistance variants in North American patients with chronic hepatitis B not receiving antiviral treatment. J Viral Hepat 2017;24(11):1032–42.

34. Smith DB, Bukh J, Kuiken C, et al. Expanded classification of hepatitis C virus into 7 genotypes and 67 subtypes: updated criteria and genotype assignment web resource. Hepatology 2014;59(1):318–27.

35. Collaborators POH. Global prevalence and genotype distribution of hepatitis C virus infection in 2015: a modelling study. Lancet Gastroenterol Hepatol 2017;2(3):161–76.

36. Westbrook RH, Dusheiko G. Natural history of hepatitis C. J Hepatol 2014;61(1 Suppl):S58–68.

37. Webster DP, Klenerman P, Dusheiko GM. Hepatitis C. Lancet 2015;385(9973):1124–35.

38. Cox AL, Netski DM, Mosbruger T, et al. Prospective evaluation of community-acquired acute-phase hepatitis C virus infection. Clin Infect Dis 2005;40(7):951–8.

39. Recommendations for prevention and control of hepatitis C virus (HCV) infection and HCV-related chronic disease. Centers for Disease Control and Prevention. MMWR Recomm Rep 1998;47(Rr-19):1–39.

40. Thomson EC, Smith JA, Klenerman P. The natural history of early hepatitis C virus evolution; lessons from a global outbreak in human immunodeficiency virus-1-infected individuals. J Gen Virol 2011;92(Pt 10):2227–36.

41. Hoofnagle JH. Hepatitis C: the clinical spectrum of disease. Hepatology 1997; 26(3 Suppl 1):15s–20s.
42. Gerlach JT, Diepolder HM, Zachoval R, et al. Acute hepatitis C: high rate of both spontaneous and treatment-induced viral clearance. Gastroenterology 2003; 125(1):80–8.
43. Frias M, Rivero-Juarez A, Rodriguez-Cano D, et al. HLA-B, HLA-C and KIR improve the predictive value of IFNL3 for Hepatitis C spontaneous clearance. Sci Rep 2018;8(1):659.
44. Beinhardt S, Payer BA, Datz C, et al. A diagnostic score for the prediction of spontaneous resolution of acute hepatitis C virus infection. J Hepatol 2013; 59(5):972–7.
45. Mondelli MU, Cerino A, Cividini A. Acute hepatitis C: diagnosis and management. J Hepatol 2005;42(Suppl 1):S108–14.
46. Marcellin P, Asselah T, Boyer N. Fibrosis and disease progression in hepatitis C. Hepatology 2002;36(5 Suppl 1):S47–56.
47. Schmidt WN, Stapleton JT, LaBrecque DR, et al. Hepatitis C virus (HCV) infection and cryoglobulinemia: analysis of whole blood and plasma HCV-RNA concentrations and correlation with liver histology. Hepatology 2000;31(3):737–44.
48. Farci P, Alter HJ, Wong D, et al. A long-term study of hepatitis C virus replication in non-A, non-B hepatitis. N Engl J Med 1991;325(2):98–104.
49. Thimme R, Bukh J, Spangenberg HC, et al. Viral and immunological determinants of hepatitis C virus clearance, persistence, and disease. Proc Natl Acad Sci U S A 2002;99(24):15661–8.
50. Pawlotsky JM. Use and interpretation of virological tests for hepatitis C. Hepatology 2002;36(5 Suppl 1):S65–73.
51. Glynn SA, Wright DJ, Kleinman SH, et al. Dynamics of viremia in early hepatitis C virus infection. Transfusion 2005;45(6):994–1002.
52. Schijman A, Colina R, Mukomolov S, et al. Comparison of hepatitis C viral loads in patients with or without coinfection with different genotypes. Clin Diagn Lab Immunol 2004;11(2):433–5.
53. Busch MP. Insights into the epidemiology, natural history and pathogenesis of hepatitis C virus infection from studies of infected donors and blood product recipients. Transfus Clin Biol 2001;8(3):200–6.
54. Netski DM, Mosbruger T, Depla E, et al. Humoral immune response in acute hepatitis C virus infection. Clin Infect Dis 2005;41(5):667–75.
55. Thomson EC, Nastouli E, Main J, et al. Delayed anti-HCV antibody response in HIV-positive men acutely infected with HCV. AIDS 2009;23(1):89–93.
56. Schmidt WN, Wu P, Cederna J, et al. Surreptitious hepatitis C virus (HCV) infection detected in the majority of patients with cryptogenic chronic hepatitis and negative HCV antibody tests. J Infect Dis 1997;176(1):27–33.
57. George SL, Gebhardt J, Klinzman D, et al. Hepatitis C virus viremia in HIV-infected individuals with negative HCV antibody tests. J Acquir Immune Defic Syndr 2002;31(2):154–62.
58. Rehermann B, Nascimbeni M. Immunology of hepatitis B virus and hepatitis C virus infection. Nat Rev Immunol 2005;5(3):215–29.
59. Bhattarai N, McLinden JH, Xiang J, et al. Hepatitis C virus infection inhibits a Src-kinase regulatory phosphatase and reduces T cell activation in vivo. PLoS Pathog 2017;13(2):e1006232.
60. Lee SR, Kardos KW, Schiff E, et al. Evaluation of a new, rapid test for detecting HCV infection, suitable for use with blood or oral fluid. J Virol Methods 2011; 172(1–2):27–31.

61. Ross RS, Viazov S, Salloum S, et al. Analytical performance characteristics and clinical utility of a novel assay for total hepatitis C virus core antigen quantification. J Clin Microbiol 2010;48(4):1161–8.

62. Tedder RS, Tuke P, Wallis N, et al. Therapy-induced clearance of HCV core antigen from plasma predicts an end of treatment viral response. J Viral Hepat 2013;20(1):65–71.

63. AASLD, IDSA. HCV guidance: recommendations for testing, managing, and treating hepatitis C 2017. Available at: https://www.hcvguidelines.org/. Accessed May 11, 2018.

64. Pawlotsky JM, Bouvier-Alias M, Hezode C, et al. Standardization of hepatitis C virus RNA quantification. Hepatology 2000;32(3):654–9.

65. Pawlotsky JM. Measuring hepatitis C viremia in clinical samples: can we trust the assays? Hepatology 1997;26(1):1–4.

66. Tobler LH, Stramer SL, Lee SR, et al. Impact of HCV 3.0 EIA relative to HCV 2.0 EIA on blood-donor screening. Transfusion 2003;43(10):1452–9.

67. Quiroga JA, Campillo ML, Catillo I, et al. IgM antibody to hepatitis C virus in acute and chronic hepatitis C. Hepatology 1991;14(1):38–43.

68. Schmidt WN, Nelson DR, Pawlotsky JM, et al. Direct-acting antiviral agents and the path to interferon independence. Clin Gastroenterol Hepatol 2014;12(5):728–37.

69. Simmonds P. Viral heterogeneity of the hepatitis C virus. J Hepatol 1999;31(Suppl 1):54–60.

70. Orland JR, Wright TL, Cooper S. Acute hepatitis C. Hepatology 2001;33(2):321–7.

71. Papastergiou V, Tsochatzis E, Burroughs AK. Non-invasive assessment of liver fibrosis. Ann Gastroenterol 2012;25(3):218–31.

72. Wang CJ, Chen PJ, Wu JC, et al. Small-form hepatitis B surface antigen is sufficient to help in the assembly of hepatitis delta virus-like particles. J Virol 1991;65(12):6630–6.

73. Le Gal F, Gault E, Ripault MP, et al. Eighth major clade for hepatitis delta virus. Emerg Infect Dis 2006;12(9):1447–50.

74. Chatzinoff M, Friedman LS. Delta agent hepatitis. Infect Dis Clin North Am 1987;1(3):529–45.

75. Yurdaydin C, Idilman R, Bozkaya H, et al. Natural history and treatment of chronic delta hepatitis. J Viral Hepat 2010;17(11):749–56.

76. Romeo R, Del Ninno E, Rumi M, et al. A 28-year study of the course of hepatitis Delta infection: a risk factor for cirrhosis and hepatocellular carcinoma. Gastroenterology 2009;136(5):1629–38.

77. Pascarella S, Negro F. Hepatitis D virus: an update. Liver Int 2011;31(1):7–21.

78. Shattock AG, Morris MC. Evaluation of commercial enzyme immunoassays for detection of hepatitis delta antigen and anti-hepatitis delta virus (HDV) and immunoglobulin M anti-HDV antibodies. J Clin Microbiol 1991;29(9):1873–6.

79. Castelnau C, Le Gal F, Ripault MP, et al. Efficacy of peginterferon alpha-2b in chronic hepatitis delta: relevance of quantitative RT-PCR for follow-up. Hepatology 2006;44(3):728–35.

80. Mederacke I, Bremer B, Heidrich B, et al. Establishment of a novel quantitative hepatitis D virus (HDV) RNA assay using the Cobas TaqMan platform to study HDV RNA kinetics. J Clin Microbiol 2010;48(6):2022–9.

81. Le Gal F, Brichler S, Sahli R, et al. First international external quality assessment for hepatitis delta virus RNA quantification in plasma. Hepatology 2016;64(5):1483–94.

82. Le Gal F, Dziri S, Gerber A, et al. Performance characteristics of a new consensus commercial kit for hepatitis D virus RNA viral load quantification. J Clin Microbiol 2017;55(2):431–41.
83. Chudy M, Hanschmann K-M, Bozdayi M, et al. Collaborative study to establish a World Health Organization international standard for hepatitis D virus RNA for nucleic acid amplification technique (NAT)-based assays. Geneva (Switzerland): Document WHO/BS/20132227 World Health Organization; 2013.
84. Smedile A, Lavarini C, Crivelli O, et al. Radioimmunoassay detection of IgM antibodies to the HBV-associated delta (delta) antigen:" clinical significance in delta infection. J Med Virol 1982;9(2):131–8.
85. Aragona M, Macagno S, Caredda F, et al. Serological response to the hepatitis delta virus in hepatitis D. Lancet 1987;1(8531):478–80.
86. Borghesio E, Rosina F, Smedile A, et al. Serum immunoglobulin M antibody to hepatitis D as a surrogate marker of hepatitis D in interferon-treated patients and in patients who underwent liver transplantation. Hepatology 1998;27(3): 873–6.
87. Hughes SA, Wedemeyer H, Harrison PM. Hepatitis delta virus. Lancet 2011; 378(9785):73–85.
88. Wedemeyer H, Yurdaydin C, Dalekos GN, et al. Peginterferon plus adefovir versus either drug alone for hepatitis delta. N Engl J Med 2011;364(4):322–31.
89. Schlauder GG, Dawson GJ, Erker JC, et al. The sequence and phylogenetic analysis of a novel hepatitis E virus isolated from a patient with acute hepatitis reported in the United States. J Gen Virol 1998;79(Pt 3):447–56.
90. Kamar N, Dalton HR, Abravanel F, et al. Hepatitis E virus infection. Clin Microbiol Rev 2014;27(1):116–38.
91. Dalton HR, Bendall R, Ijaz S, et al. Hepatitis E: an emerging infection in developed countries. Lancet Infect Dis 2008;8(11):698–709.
92. Dalton HR, Bendall RP, Keane FE, et al. Persistent carriage of hepatitis E virus in patients with HIV infection. N Engl J Med 2009;361(10):1025–7.
93. Gerolami R, Moal V, Picard C, et al. Hepatitis E virus as an emerging cause of chronic liver disease in organ transplant recipients. J Hepatol 2009;50(3):622–4.
94. Kamar N, Mansuy JM, Cointault O, et al. Hepatitis E virus-related cirrhosis in kidney- and kidney-pancreas-transplant recipients. Am J Transplant 2008;8(8): 1744–8.
95. Aggarwal R, Kini D, Sofat S, et al. Duration of viraemia and faecal viral excretion in acute hepatitis E. Lancet 2000;356(9235):1081–2.
96. Huang S, Zhang X, Jiang H, et al. Profile of acute infectious markers in sporadic hepatitis E. PLoS One 2010;5(10):e13560.
97. Kamar N, Rostaing L, Legrand-Abravanel F, et al. How should hepatitis E virus infection be defined in organ-transplant recipients? Am J Transplant 2013;13(7): 1935–6.
98. Drobeniuc J, Meng J, Reuter G, et al. Serologic assays specific to immunoglobulin M antibodies against hepatitis E virus: pangenotypic evaluation of performances. Clin Infect Dis 2010;51(3):e24–7.
99. Yoo N, Bernstein J, Caldwell C, et al. Hepatitis E virus infection in a liver transplant recipient: delayed diagnosis due to variable performance of serologic assays. Transpl Infect Dis 2013;15(4):E166–8.
100. Sue PK, Pisanic N, Heaney CD, et al. Variability of hepatitis E serologic assays in a pediatric liver transplant recipient: challenges to diagnosing hepatitis E virus infection in the United States. Transpl Infect Dis 2015;17(2):284–8.

Liver Fibrosis Determination

Michelle Lai, MD, MPH*, Nezam H. Afdhal, MD

KEYWORDS

- Liver fibrosis • NAFLD fibrosis score • FIB-4 • APRI • Hepascore • Fibrotest
- Fibrosure • ELF

KEY POINTS

- All chronic liver diseases can lead to liver fibrosis.
- Liver fibrosis determination is important for determining prognosis and making treatment and management decisions in all chronic liver diseases.
- Radiologic liver fibrosis determinations are increasingly used but are not as widely available as laboratory liver fibrosis determinations.
- Laboratory liver fibrosis determinations include general clinical scoring systems and commercially available combination biomarker panels.
- Laboratory liver fibrosis determinations are useful for assessing whether a patient is at low, intermediate, or high risk of advanced fibrosis and eliminating the need for liver biopsy in a substantial proportion of patients.

INTRODUCTION

Chronic liver disease is a significant problem in the United States and worldwide (**Fig. 1, Tables 1** and **2**). In the United States, 3.5 million Americans have chronic hepatitis C, up to 2.2 million Americans have chronic hepatitis B, and an estimated 64 million have nonalcoholic fatty liver disease (NAFLD).[1–3] All of these chronic liver diseases can lead to liver fibrosis with progression to cirrhosis. Advanced liver fibrosis and cirrhosis are associated with liver-related mortality, including liver failure and hepatocellular carcinoma. An estimated 5 million Americans are estimated to have advanced fibrosis from NAFLD alone.[4] Assessment of fibrosis severity provides prognostic value and is vital to making treatment and management decisions. Patients with significant fibrosis should be treated more urgently to prevent progression to cirrhosis, whereas patients with advanced fibrosis should also be regularly screened for varices and hepatocellular carcinoma.

Disclosure Statement: Dr N.H. Afdhal is a consultant for Echosens. Dr M. Lai has nothing to disclose.
Department of Medicine, Liver Center, Beth Israel Deaconess Medical Center, Harvard Medical School, 110 Francis Street, Suite 4A, Boston, MA 02215, USA
* Corresponding author.
E-mail address: mlai@bidmc.harvard.edu

Gastroenterol Clin N Am 48 (2019) 281–289
https://doi.org/10.1016/j.gtc.2019.02.002
0889-8553/19/© 2019 Elsevier Inc. All rights reserved.

gastro.theclinics.com

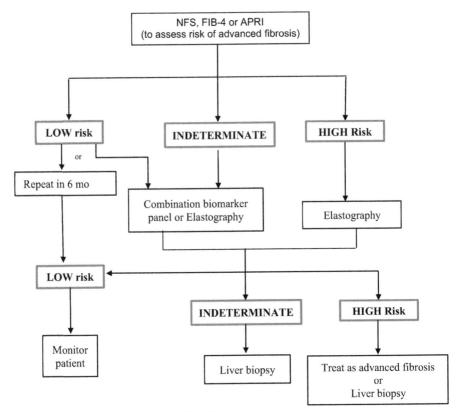

Fig. 1. Liver fibrosis determination flowchart.

Although the gold standard for fibrosis assessment is a liver biopsy, its well-known limitations have made it unattractive to clinicians and patients. However, this is an invasive procedure with potential complications, such as pain (20%) and bleeding (0.5%).[5] In addition to the potential complications, it is also limited by sampling errors and intraobserver and interobserver variations. Because liver biopsies only sample an extremely small portion of the liver (1/50,000), sampling errors can occur.[5] Histologic examination is also prone to intraobserver and interobserver variations. Because of these limitations of liver biopsy, many noninvasive liver fibrosis assessment tools have been developed to decrease the need for a liver biopsy in most patients. Imaging tests, such as transient elastography and MR elastography, are increasingly used for fibrosis assessment and have been able to eliminate the need for liver biopsy in up to 70% of patients, particularly with viral hepatitis. However, the availability of these imaging modalities is limited to certain clinical settings given the cost and the requirement for the upfront capital investment.

Laboratory-based liver fibrosis determination is widely available and accessible to all clinicians. In this article, the authors discuss the most commonly used general clinical scoring systems and combination biomarker panels.

GENERAL CLINICAL SCORING SYSTEMS

General clinical scoring systems are based on readily available clinical and laboratory variables as well as published formulas. Three commonly used systems are the

Table 1
General clinical scoring systems and cutoffs for advanced fibrosis

	Risk Category	NFS[6,7]	FIB4[8–10]	APRI[11–13]
Variables		Age, BMI, hyperglycemia, platelet count, albumin, AST/ALT ratio)	Platelet count, age, AST, ALT	AST, platelet count
Formula		$-1.675 + 0.037 \times$ age (y) $+ 0.094 \times$ BMI (kg/m^2) $+ 1.13 \times$ IFG/ diabetes (yes $= 1$, no $= 0$) $+ 0.99 \times$ AST/ ALT ratio $- 0.013 \times$ platelet ($\times 10^9$/L) $- 0.66 \times$ albumin (g/dL)	(Age $\times$ AST)/(Platelets $\times$ (sqr (ALT)))	[(AST/ULN AST) $\times$ 100]/ platelets (10^9/L)]
Cutoffs in NAFLD	Low risk	< -1.455 (NPV = 88%)	<1.30 (NPV = 90%)	≤1.0 (NPV = 84%)
	Indeterminate	-1.455–0.675	1.30–3.25	
	High risk	>0.675 (PPV = 82%)	>2.67 (PPV = 80%)	>1.0 (PPV = 37%)
AUROC		0.82–0.85	0.80	0.67
Cutoffs in HCV	Low risk		<1.45 (NPV = 90%)	≤1.0[a] (NPV = 100%)
	Indeterminate		1.45–3.25	1.0–2.0[a]
	High risk		>3.25 (PPV = 65%) >5.88[a] (PPV = 82.5%)	>2.0[a] (PPV = 65%)
AUROC			0.765–0.83	0.94
Cutoffs in HBV	Low risk		<1.58 (NPV = 84.6%)	≤1.0–1.5[a] (NPV = 86%)
	Indeterminate		1.58–5.17	
	High risk		>5.17[a] (PPV = 83.3%)	>1.0–1.5[a] (PPV = 39%)
AUROC			0.845	0.75

[a] Cutoff for cirrhosis.

NAFLD Fibrosis Score (NFS), Fibrosis-4 (FIB-4), and the aspartate aminotransferase (AST) to Platelet Ratio Index (APRI). These 3 scoring systems all have a cutoff value below which the patient is deemed to be low risk for significant fibrosis (Kleiner or Metavir F0-2), advanced fibrosis (F3-4), or cirrhosis (F4). They also have a second cutoff above which the patient is deemed high risk. If the score falls between these 2 cutoffs, the result is indeterminate.

Nonalcoholic Fatty Liver Disease Fibrosis Score

The NFS is a disease-specific scoring system used in patients with NAFLD and is based on 6 variables (age, body mass index [BMI], hyperglycemia, platelet count, albumin, and AST/alanine aminotransferase [ALT] ratio). A score less than

Table 2
Combination biomarker panels

	Risk Category	ELF[14–16]	Hepascore (Liver Fibrosis Panel)[18–20]	Fibrotest (FibroSure)[21–24]
Variables		Hyaluronic acid, tissue inhibitor of metalloproteinase 1, N-terminal procollagen III peptide	Age, sex, α2-macroglobulin, gamma-glutamyl transpeptidase, bilirubin, hyaluronic acid	Age, sex, α2-macroglobulin, gamma-glutamyl transpeptidase, bilirubin, haptoglobin, apolipoprotein A1
NAFLD	Cutoff	10.35 (NPV = 94%)	0.37 (NPV = 97%)	0.30 (NPV = 97%)
	AUROC	0.90	0.81	0.88
HCV	Cutoff	0.063 (NPV = 95%)	0.47 (NPV = 95%)	0.52 (NPV = 94%)
	AUROC	0.773	0.86	0.84
HBV	Cutoff	8.4 (NPV = 88%)	0.42 (NPV = 90%)	0.48 (NPV = 90%)
	AUROC	0.69	0.82	0.82

−1.455 predicts no advanced fibrosis; a score greater than 0.675 predicts advanced fibrosis, and a score in between (−1.455–0.675, inclusive) is considered indeterminate. Advanced fibrosis was defined as stage 3 to 4 fibrosis on the Kleiner scoring system. The area under the receiver operating characteristic curve (AUROC) was 0.88 and 0.82 in the estimation and validation groups, respectively.[6] In a meta-analysis of 13 studies with 3064 patients, the NFS had an AUROC of 0.85 for predicting advanced fibrosis.[7] About a quarter (28%) of patients were indeterminate.[6]

Fibrosis-4 Index

FIB-4 index is another clinical scoring system that, as its name suggests, is based on 4 variables (platelet count, age, AST, and ALT). It also gives a score that is either low risk for advanced fibrosis (<1.45), high risk for advanced fibrosis (>3.25), or indeterminate (1.45–3.25, inclusive). It was originally derived in an human immunodeficiency virus (HIV)/hepatitis C virus (HCV) coinfected cohort of patients and looked at those cutoffs for predicting advanced fibrosis (Ishak ≥4).[8] Validation of FIB-4 using the low risk cutoff of <1.45 and high risk cutoff of >3.25 in a larger cohort of 2304 monoinfected HCV patients from the Chronic Hepatitis Cohort Study to predict cirrhosis and rule out advanced fibrosis.[9] This study found that an FIB-4 ≤1.21 ruled out advanced fibrosis with 92.7% negative predictive value (NPV). On the other end of the disease spectrum, an FIB-4 greater than 5.88 had an 82.5% positive prediction value for cirrhosis. These cutoffs gave an AUROC of 0.83. In this same cohort, 284 patients with chronic hepatitis B virus (HBV) were analyzed. An FIB-4 index of ≤1.58 ruled out advanced fibrosis with 84.6% NPV and an FIB-4 index of greater than 5.17 predicted cirrhosis with 83.3% positive predictive value (PPV). Using these cutoffs, the AUROC was 0.86.

Another study with 541 patients validated the use of FIB-4 in NAFLD patients, albeit with different ideal cutoffs, to predict advanced fibrosis.[10] An FIB-4 index ≥2.67 had an 80% PPV, whereas an FIB-4 index ≤1.30 had a 90% NPV, overall giving an AUROC of 0.802, with 30% of the patient with an indeterminate score.

Aspartate Aminotransferase to Platelet Ratio Index

APRI is a simple formula based on the 2 commonly available clinical variables that are also used in both NFS and FIB-4, the AST and platelet count. It was developed using a cohort of patients with HCV to predict significant fibrosis or cirrhosis to help with treatment decisions during the era of interferon-based therapy.[11] Currently, with the availability of directly acting antiviral therapies with minimal side effects and high cure rates, the distinction between significant fibrosis and minimal fibrosis is less relevant. However, the diagnosis of cirrhosis is still important to management because the clinician needs to know whether to screen for hepatocellular carcinoma and varices even if the virus is eradicated. In the validation cohort of this original study, the NPV for an APRI ≤1.0 was excellent at 100%. The PPV of an APRI greater than 2.0 for predicting cirrhosis was 65%. In other words, this is a good test for "ruling out" cirrhosis, but values in the indeterminate range or greater than 2.00 requires biopsy for more accurate staging unless there are other clinical features of cirrhosis.

A meta-analysis that included data from 6 studies with a total of 1012 patients assessed the performance of APRI in patients with chronic hepatitis B infection.[12] For the prediction of significant fibrosis (F2-4), the AUROC was 0.79 with sensitivity, specificity, PPV, and NPV of 84%, 41%, 64%, and 68%, respectively, for the cutoff of 0.5. A cutoff of 1.5 was less sensitive (49%) and more specific, giving a PPV of 80% and an NPV of 57%. In this same meta-analysis, the summary AUROC was 0.75 for the prediction of cirrhosis with sensitivity, specificity, PPV, and NPV of 54%, 78%, 39%, and 86%, respectively, for cutoffs 1.0 to 1.5. Raising the cutoff to 2.0 decreased the sensitivity to 28%, increased the specificity (87%), giving a PPV of 36% and NPV of 87%.

The validation of APRI in a cohort of 145 patients with NAFLD for detection of advanced fibrosis using the cutoff of 1.0 gave a low sensitivity of 27% with a specificity of 89%.[13] The AUROC dropped below that of NFS and FIB-4 at 0.67.

The appeal of these 3 general clinical scoring systems is that they are based on readily available clinical variables using a free publicly available formula. At the time of the visit, the clinician can make a quick calculation based on the most recent laboratory tests available to quickly assess whether the patient is at low or high risk of having advanced fibrosis and determine whether further assessment such as a liver biopsy is necessary. The reduction from 4 to 6 variables (NFS and FIB-4) to 2 (APRI) variables results in the reduction in the AUROC.

The authors recommend utilizing these simple tests in the following way as the initial screening;

1. Low risk: Unlikely for advanced fibrosis, follow patient and repeat in 6 months or confirm with combination biomarker panel or fibrosis imaging.
2. Indeterminate score: Suggest combination biomarker test or an imaging test, such as ultrasound elastography (FibroScan). If again indeterminate, consider liver biopsy.
3. High risk: Confirm with elastography, and if confirmed, treat as advanced liver disease or consider liver biopsy.

COMBINATION BIOMARKER PANELS

Three commonly used commercially available blood-based algorithms to predict fibrosis are the enhanced liver fibrosis (ELF) panel, Fibrotest (Fibrosure), and Hepascore, which are good tests for the prediction of advanced fibrosis with AUROC ranging between 0.81 and 0.90.

Enhanced Liver Fibrosis

The ELF panel is a blood-based algorithm developed by the European Liver Fibrosis Group consisting of the plasma levels of 3 matrix turnover proteins (hyaluronic acid, tissue inhibitor of metalloproteinase 1, and N-terminal procollagen III peptide). The original study by the group developed the OELF (Original ELF), which included age in the algorithm along with the plasma levels of the 3 proteins in a cohort of 1021 patients with various chronic liver diseases.[14] An updated panel (ELF) was presented after a validation study showed that the test accuracy was not reduced by leaving out age in the algorithm in a cohort of NAFLD patients.[15] In this validation cohort, the ELF panel had excellent performance in distinguishing advanced fibrosis in patients with NAFLD with an AUROC of 0.90. However, it was shown that the test performance can be affected by gender and age in patients with chronic hepatitis C.[16] There are less data on the use of ELF in chronic hepatitis B, but the performance does not appear to be as good, with an AUROC of 0.67.[17]

Hepascore and Fibrotest (known as FibroSure in the United States) are 2 other blood-based algorithms that also include age and sex. In addition to age and sex, they have 3 serum parameters in common: α2-macroglobulin, gamma-glutamyl transpeptidase, and bilirubin.

Hepascore

Hepascore combines clinical variables of age and gender with blood-based parameters, including bilirubin, gamma-glutamyl transferase, hyaluronic acid, and α2-macroglobulin.[18] It was initially developed in patients with chronic hepatitis C and shown to be excellent at excluding advanced fibrosis with a cutoff of less than 0.5.[18] In a prospective study evaluating the performance of laboratory-based algorithms in excluding advanced fibrosis in patients with chronic hepatitis B and chronic hepatitis C, the optimal cutoff differed by disease.[19] The ideal cutoff for chronic hepatitis B was 0.48 and 0.52 for HCV. When studied in patients with NAFLD, a cutoff of 0.37 was better at identifying individuals with advanced fibrosis.[20]

FibroTest

FibroTest (known as FibroSure in the United States) was initially validated in patients with chronic hepatitis C, but has since been validated in other liver disease, including HBV and NAFLD.[21–24] In addition to the variables shared with Hepascore (age, sex, α2-macroglobulin, gamma-glutamyl transpeptidase, and bilirubin), it also includes haptoglobin and apolipoprotein A1. It performs well across the different liver diseases with AUROC ranging from 0.82 to 0.88. Its diagnostic performance may be reduced with acute inflammation, sepsis, and extrahepatic cholestasis.[22]

All of these commercially available laboratory-based combination biomarker panels have excellent NPV in ruling out advanced fibrosis in chronic liver diseases. Although ELF is used widely in Europe, it is not available in the United States, where Hepascore and Fibrotest (FibroSure) are mainly used.

DISCUSSION

These widely available noninvasive laboratory liver fibrosis assessment tools have revolutionized the management of patients with chronic liver diseases. They have decreased the need for the invasive liver biopsy in a large proportion of patients. The scoring systems also have prognostic values in predicting future liver-related outcomes.[25] The cutoffs for general clinical scoring systems vary depending on the cause of liver disease and whether one is trying to predict significant fibrosis, advanced fibrosis, or cirrhosis. The answer asked by the clinician as to whether the patient has significant fibrosis, advanced fibrosis, or cirrhosis depends on the clinical context and how it would change management. For example, in patients with NALFD, advanced fibrosis predicts liver-related mortality. The presence of advanced fibrosis from nonalcoholic steatohepatitis would warrant the initiation of screening for hepatocellular carcinoma and varices as well as consideration for referral to bariatric surgery and consideration for clinical trial or pharmacologic treatment once they become available. In this current era of multiple directly acting antiviral regimens for the treatment of chronic hepatitis C, all patients with chronic hepatitis C should be considered for treatment regardless of stage of fibrosis. However, the presence of cirrhosis could change the treatment regimen. Also, in patients with chronic hepatitis C who have achieved sustained virologic response, liver fibrosis assessment suggesting cirrhosis would require that the patient continue screening for hepatocellular carcinoma and varices. Significant fibrosis in patients with chronic hepatitis B would make a case for starting the patient on antiviral treatment. The presence of advanced fibrosis or cirrhosis would warrant regular screening for hepatocellular carcinoma.

What these markers have in common are excellent NPVs for ruling out advanced fibrosis. Patients with indeterminate, intermediate, or high-risk scores should be considered for liver biopsy if the results would change management. As with all tests, the results should be interpreted in the clinical context. For example, a patient with Gilbert or with indirect hyperbilirubinemia from HIV antiretroviral treatment will have a higher Hepascore or Fibrotest that is not an accurate reflection of their fibrosis stage because total bilirubin is part of the algorithm. Knowing the variables that are part of these liver fibrosis determination tools and their test performance allows for valuable clinical application of these tools.

These study cohorts in which the biomarkers and scoring systems were developed and validated consist of patients with a single liver disease. However, in the general population, many patients have more than 1 liver disease. With the prevalence of NAFLD estimated in up to one-third of the general population, many patients with chronic hepatitis B or chronic hepatitis C infections also have concurrent NAFLD. Because the cutoffs may differ by disease, this complicates the interpretation of the results. In the absence of substantial data on the optimal cutoffs in these patients, the authors recommend using a lower cutoff to avoid missing advanced fibrosis. The use of a lower cutoff would come at a cost of more liver biopsies. In those with NAFLD and HCV with an intermediate cutoff, one approach could be to repeat the liver fibrosis determination after sustained virologic response. In those with NAFLD and HBV, a liver biopsy may also give information on the pattern of inflammation to see if NAFLD or HBV is the main driving force of liver fibrosis.

REFERENCES

1. Younossi ZM, Blissett D, Blissett R, et al. The economic and clinical burden of nonalcoholic fatty liver disease in the United States and Europe. Hepatology 2016;64(5):1577–86.
2. Edlin BR, Eckhardt BJ, Shu MA, et al. Toward a more accurate estimate of the prevalence of hepatitis C in the United States. Hepatology 2015;62(5): 1353–63.
3. Kowdley KV, Wang CC, Welch S, et al. Prevalence of chronic hepatitis B among foreign-born persons living in the United States by country of origin. Hepatology 2012;56(2):422–33.
4. Wong RJ, Liu B, Bhuket T. Significant burden of nonalcoholic fatty liver disease with advanced fibrosis in the US: a cross-sectional analysis of 2011-2014 National Health and Nutrition Examination Survey. Aliment Pharmacol Ther 2017; 46(10):974–80.

5. Bedossa P, Dargere D, Paradis V. Sampling variability of liver fibrosis in chronic hepatitis C. Hepatology 2003;38(6):1449–57.

6. Angulo P, Hui JM, Marchesini G, et al. The NAFLD fibrosis score: a noninvasive system that identifies liver fibrosis in patients with NAFLD. Hepatology 2007; 45(4):846–54.

7. Musso G, Gambino R, Cassader M, et al. Meta-analysis: natural history of non-alcoholic fatty liver disease (NAFLD) and diagnostic accuracy of non-invasive tests for liver disease severity. Ann Med 2011;43(8):617–49.

8. Sterling RK, Lissen E, Clumeck N, et al. Development of a simple noninvasive index to predict significant fibrosis in patients with HIV/HCV coinfection. Hepatology 2006;43(6):1317–25.

9. Li J, Gordon SC, Rupp LB, et al. The validity of serum markers for fibrosis staging in chronic hepatitis B and C. J Viral Hepat 2014;21(12):930–7.

10. Shah AG, Lydecker A, Murray K, et al. Comparison of noninvasive markers of fibrosis in patients with nonalcoholic fatty liver disease. Clin Gastroenterol Hepatol 2009;7(10):1104–12.

11. Wai CT, Greenson JK, Fontana RJ, et al. A simple noninvasive index can predict both significant fibrosis and cirrhosis in patients with chronic hepatitis C. Hepatology 2003;38(2):518–26.

12. Jin W, Lin Z, Xin Y, et al. Diagnostic accuracy of the aspartate aminotransferase-to-platelet ratio index for the prediction of hepatitis B-related fibrosis: a leading meta-analysis. BMC Gastroenterol 2012;12:14.

13. McPherson S, Stewart SF, Henderson E, et al. Simple non-invasive fibrosis scoring systems can reliably exclude advanced fibrosis in patients with nonalcoholic fatty liver disease. Gut 2010;59(9):1265–9.

14. Rosenberg WM, Voelker M, Thiel R, et al. Serum markers detect the presence of liver fibrosis: a cohort study. Gastroenterology 2004;127(6):1704–13.

15. Guha IN, Parkes J, Roderick P, et al. Noninvasive markers of fibrosis in nonalcoholic fatty liver disease: Validating the European Liver Fibrosis Panel and exploring simple markers. Hepatology 2008;47(2):455–60.

16. Lichtinghagen R, Pietsch D, Bantel H, et al. The Enhanced Liver Fibrosis (ELF) score: normal values, influence factors and proposed cut-off values. J Hepatol 2013;59(2):236–42.

17. Wong GL, Chan HL, Choi PC, et al. Non-invasive algorithm of enhanced liver fibrosis and liver stiffness measurement with transient elastography for advanced liver fibrosis in chronic hepatitis B. Aliment Pharmacol Ther 2014;39(2):197–208.

18. Adams LA, Bulsara M, Rossi E, et al. Hepascore: an accurate validated predictor of liver fibrosis in chronic hepatitis C infection. Clin Chem 2005;51(10):1867–73.

19. Leroy V, Sturm N, Faure P, et al. Prospective evaluation of FibroTest(R), FibroMeter(R), and HepaScore(R) for staging liver fibrosis in chronic hepatitis B: comparison with hepatitis C. J Hepatol 2014;61(1):28–34.

20. Adams LA, George J, Bugianesi E, et al. Complex non-invasive fibrosis models are more accurate than simple models in non-alcoholic fatty liver disease. J Gastroenterol Hepatol 2011;26(10):1536–43.

21. Poynard T, Imbert-Bismut F, Munteanu M, et al. Overview of the diagnostic value of biochemical markers of liver fibrosis (FibroTest, HCV FibroSure) and necrosis (ActiTest) in patients with chronic hepatitis C. Comp Hepatol 2004;3(1):8.

22. Poynard T, Morra R, Halfon P, et al. Meta-analyses of FibroTest diagnostic value in chronic liver disease. BMC Gastroenterol 2007;7:40.

23. Poynard T, Zoulim F, Ratziu V, et al. Longitudinal assessment of histology surrogate markers (FibroTest-ActiTest) during lamivudine therapy in patients with chronic hepatitis B infection. Am J Gastroenterol 2005;100(9):1970–80.
24. Ratziu V, Massard J, Charlotte F, et al. Diagnostic value of biochemical markers (FibroTest-FibroSURE) for the prediction of liver fibrosis in patients with nonalcoholic fatty liver disease. BMC Gastroenterol 2006;6:6.
25. Angulo P, Bugianesi E, Bjornsson ES, et al. Simple noninvasive systems predict long-term outcomes of patients with nonalcoholic fatty liver disease. Gastroenterology 2013;145(4):782–9.e4.

IgG4-Related Disease with Emphasis on Its Gastrointestinal Manifestation

Bijal Vashi, MD[a], Arezou Khosroshahi, MD[b],*

KEYWORDS

- IgG4-RD • IgG4 • Autoimmune pancreatitis • Cholangitis • Rituximab

KEY POINTS

- In IgG4-RD, organs can be synchronously or metachronously affected, leading to clinical and diagnostic ambiguity.
- Clinical histopathologic findings are the gold standard for confirmation of diagnosis.
- The most common gastrointestinal organs involved by IgG4-RD are the pancreas and bile ducts, although most cases have other organ involvement at the time of diagnosis.
- Glucocorticoids are the best induction therapy, although disease relapse is common.
- Rituximab has shown promise as steroid-sparing therapy for IgG4-RD.

INTRODUCTION

IgG4-related disease (IgG4-RD) is a multisystem immune-mediated fibroinflammatory condition with a wide spectrum of organ system involvement that can be synchronous at the time of diagnosis or be metachronous over the patient's lifetime.

This disease was first described in the pancreas in 1991 by Kawaguchi and colleagues[1] on resected tissue from a patient with mass-forming pancreatitis. The unusual histopathologic finding of the mass was described as lymphoplasmacytic sclerosing pancreatitis. In 1995, Yoshida and colleagues[2] proposed the term autoimmune pancreatitis (AIP) for this peculiar steroid-responsive chronic pancreatitis. Six years later, Hamano and colleagues[3] found that patients with AIP have increased serum IgG4 concentrations. Dr Kamisawa's group in Japan proposed the new clinicopathologic systemic condition of IgG4-related systemic disease in 2003, based on the observation that fibroinflammatory lesions with IgG4-producing cells can affect other

Disclosure Statement: No disclosures.
[a] Department of Medicine, Emory University, 200 Whitehead Building, 615 Michael Street, Atlanta, GA 30322, USA; [b] Department of Medicine, Emory University, 244 Whitehead Building, 615 Michael Street, Atlanta, GA 30322, USA
* Corresponding author.
E-mail address: akhosroshahi@emory.edu

gastro.theclinics.com

organ systems that were similar if not identical in the patients with AIP.[4] Their group suggested that AIP is not a type of pancreatitis but rather a pancreatic manifestation of a systemic disease. Dozens of terminologies were used until 2011 when the expert consensus declared IgG4-RD as the official name for this condition.[5] In the last decade, involvement of nearly every organ system has been described in these patients, unifying many conditions previously deemed isolated single-organ diseases.[6,7]

The mass lesions containing IgG4-producing plasma cells, lymphocytes, and fibrosis can mimic infectious, malignant, and other inflammatory causes that can make the diagnostic processes challenging. The challenge is understandable, given the tumefactive appearance on imaging in multiple sites and lack of a reliable biomarker, making tissue confirmation where possible the gold standard for diagnostic purposes.[8] Furthermore, the type and frequency of organ involvement reported typically depends on the patient's presenting symptom and the subspecialty evaluating the patient, for example, AIP or cholangitis by a gastroenterologist, or tubulointerstitial nephritis by a nephrologist.[9]

This relapsing and remitting systemic condition is clinically characterized by presence of mass-forming lesions, frequently increased serum IgG4 concentration and prompt response to glucocorticoid treatment.

In this review, we aim to discuss the key gastrointestinal manifestations of IgG4-RD for the practicing gastroenterologist and address the pathology characteristics, disease mechanism, and current recommendations for therapy.

EPIDEMIOLOGY

The epidemiology of IgG4-RD is not well understood because of the under recognition of the condition until recently. A Japanese nationwide survey indicated an overall prevalence of 4.6 per 100,000 people and an incidence of 1.4 per 100,000 people for AIP.[10] However, the fact that AIP is only one manifestation of a multiorgan disease, this number is certainly an underestimation of IgG4-RD prevalence. Multiple registries of patients with AIP and IgG4-RD demonstrated that this condition is more common in elderly men with average age of 66 years.[11–13] The male predilection is unusual for classic autoimmune diseases, for which female patients usually outnumber male patients. Head and neck involvement—the orbits, salivary glands, and sinuses—has been reported to be roughly equal in male and female patients.[13]

MECHANISM OF DISEASE

The pathogenesis of IgG4-RD is not completely understood. The evidence that there is specific histopathologic features shared by different unrelated organs, response to steroid treatment, and increased immunoglobulin levels suggests a possible antigen-driven inflammatory condition ultimately causing fibrosis in the tissues.

B cell depletion therapy with rituximab has shown significant clinical improvement in patients with IgG4-RD, supporting a central pathogenic role of B lymphocytes in this condition.[14–17] Interestingly, flow cytometry study of patients with active IgG4-RD shows an increased number of IgG4 B cells and plasmablasts.

Plasmablasts can circulate for prolonged periods in the setting of chronic antigenic stimulation or autoimmune diseases, as in patients with active systemic lupus erythematosus, but are generally present in only low concentrations in the blood of healthy individuals.[18] Of note, plasmablasts expanded in patients with IgG4-RD decrease promptly after rituximab therapy and re-emerges during the flare after therapy, correlating with disease activity.[19] Although we have not been able to prove the role for IgG4 antibody as a pathogenic antibody in IgG4-RD, IgG4+ B cells and plasmablasts have been suggested to play a major role in the pathogenesis of IgG4-RD either directly through autoantibody production or indirectly as antigen-presenting cells by activation of pathogenic CD4+ T cells.

A recent study[20] in the Netherlands suggests an increased number of patients with IgG4-RD have had exposures to occupational antigens, including solvents and metal dusts during their lifetime. These exposures are a potential explanation of the oligoclonal expansion of IgG4-switched B cells and plasmablasts that are similar to the mechanism of increased serum IgG4 levels in beekeepers.

Most lymphocytes present in the affected tissues of patients with IgG4-RD are T lymphocytes. Multiple studies have demonstrated the involvement of follicular helper T2 lymphocytes and CD4+ cytotoxic T lymphocytes in the pathogenesis of this disease.[21–23] Activation of these specific dysregulated T lymphocytes leads to production of profibrotic cytokines, which will crosstalk with B cells in these patients and lead to expansion of plasma blasts and IgG4 class -switching due to predominant helper T2 cytokines.[24]

CLINICAL MANIFESTATIONS

Any organ system in the body can be affected by IgG4-RD. Constitutional symptoms of fever and weight loss are rare in this condition. Miyabe and colleagues[25] analyzed the frequency of organ involvement in patients with IgG4-RD in 5 large series (total 758 patients).[11–13,26,27] This pooled analysis showed more than half of patients with documented IgG4-RD had 2 or more organs involved. Eighty-five percent of the organ manifestations were limited to the following 7 organs: pancreas, bile ducts, salivary glands, lacrimal glands, kidneys, retroperitoneum, and lungs. The lymph nodes were not counted toward IgG4 organ involvement. The pancreas was involved in 45% of patients; the lacrimal and salivary glands were each involved in 25% of patients, the bile ducts in 20%. and the retroperitoneum, lungs, and kidneys each in 15%. Most investigators collecting data for these 5 cohorts were gastroenterologists, which could partly explain the greater frequency of pancreas involvement.

Gastrointestinal Manifestations

The most common gastrointestinal organs affected by IgG4-RD are the pancreas followed by bile ducts. However, involvement of the liver, gallbladder, stomach, small and large intestine, and mesentery has been reported.

Autoimmune pancreatitis

Autoimmune pancreatitis was the first described manifestation of IgG4-RD and has been studied more than other manifestations of this condition. Patients with AIP usually present with painless jaundice or an imaging finding of focal pancreatic mass or diffuse swelling of the pancreas without jaundice. Development of endocrine and exocrine pancreatic insufficiency presenting with hyperglycemia and steatorrhea is not uncommon among patients with AIP. Acute painful pancreatitis is an uncommon presentation of IgG4-related AIP and other causes should be investigated thoroughly in those cases.

Main radiologic findings suggestive and at times diagnostic for AIP can be summarized as diffusely enlarged pancreas with featureless borders called sausage-shape pancreas (**Fig. 1**A) and delayed enhancement with or without a capsulelike rim on abdominal computed tomography (CT) or MRI. Findings of a focal pancreatic mass or ductal dilatation are common presentations of AIP, although it is imperative to recall that AIP is less common than pancreatic cancer, and any imaging suggestive of cancer should be thoroughly investigated for malignancy before concluding another

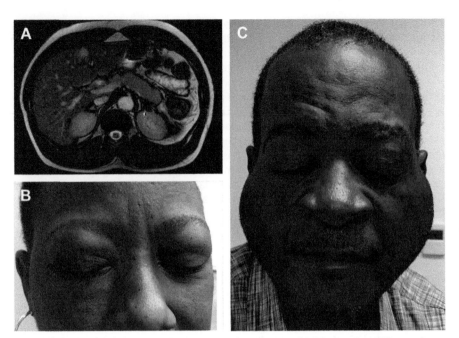

Fig. 1. Clinical features (*A*) MRI of a patient with systemic IgG4-RD showing diffuse enlargement of the pancreas; sausage-shaped pancreas. (*B*) Dacryoadenitis in a patient with IgG4-RD. (*C*) Bilateral enlargement of parotids, lacrimal glands, and submandibular glands in a patient with AIP. (Images used with subjects' consent under Emory University IRB approval no. 000–65485.)

diagnosis. Typical features on endoscopic retrograde cholangiopancreatography are diffuse narrowing of the pancreatic duct and multiple intrahepatic strictures resembling primary sclerosing cholangitis in cases associated with cholangitis.

Patients with AIP have a striking response to steroid treatment, which has been one of the diagnostic features in the HISORt (histology, imaging, serology, other organ involvement, and response to therapy) criteria for diagnosis of AIP.[28] Pancreatic experts who developed the HISORt criteria strongly discourage using a trial of steroids in the absence of other evidence and definitive histology, only to distinguish between AIP and pancreatic adenocarcinoma.[29] Patients who remain untreated or have longstanding AIP can develop features of chronic pancreatitis with atrophic pancreas and intraductal calcifications on imaging.

Key to the practicing gastroenterologist is the recognition of 2 distinct disorders of AIP. Type 1 AIP or lymphoplasmacytic sclerosing pancreatitis, also called IgG4-related pancreatitis, demonstrates the classic histology of IgG4-RD with lymphoplasmacytic infiltrate with increased IgG4+ plasma cells. This finding is an important distinction from type 2 AIP or idiopathic duct-centric pancreatitis (IDCP) marked by neutrophilic infiltrates and occasionally epithelioid granulomas in the ducts, findings of which are generally conflicting with the established consensus on pathology of IgG4-RD.[30,31]

In contrast to IgG4-related AIP, patients with IDCP tend to be younger, with a mean age of about 40 years and a male to female ratio of 1:1. Patients with IDCP tend to present mostly with recurrent acute pancreatitis in more than half of patients. Painless obstructive jaundice with a focal pancreatic mass are rare manifestation of IDCP.

Extrapancreatic involvement that is a characteristic of IgG4-related AIP is not present in IDCP, which is strongly associated with inflammatory bowel disease (mostly ulcerative colitis).[32]

Cholangitis

The most common manifestation of IgG4 cholangitis is obstructive jaundice or asymptomatic increase of liver enzymes. Evaluation can be performed with different imaging modalities including CT, MRI, magnetic resonance cholangiopancreatography, or endoscopic retrograde cholangiopancreatography and will characteristically demonstrate strictures and narrowing of the bile ducts, resembling those of primary sclerosing cholangitis (PSC) and cholangiocarcinoma.[33,34] These strictures are long segments and smooth in morphology, with resultant proximal biliary tree dilatation. Bile duct wall thickening is apparent on cross-sectional imaging and will have enhancement on postcontrast imaging series. The most common area of involvement is at the intrapancreatic segment of the common bile duct, although both the intrahepatic and extrahepatic bile ducts can be affected.[35,36]

These findings are similar to the differential diagnosis of PSC, which in contrast usually affects a younger patient demographic and has multifocal short-segment strictures, leading to the classic description of a "beaded" appearance on imaging.[37] Neither serum IgG4 concentrations nor cholangiographic or cholangioscopic findings can definitely differentiate these disorders. Therefore, endoscopic transpapillary biopsy is generally recommended. Usually, the biopsy is useful for excluding cholangiocarcinoma, but there is much debate among experts about its usefulness for the diagnosis of IgG4-related sclerosing cholangitis and PSC.[38,39]

As with the pancreatic and other extrapancreatic findings of IgG4-RD, IgG4 cholangitis has a good response to therapy with corticosteroids. Posttreatment imaging will reflect radiologic improvement in strictures and biliary tree wall thickening.[40]

Cholecystitis

In addition to the biliary tree itself, the gallbladder wall can be thickened by IgG4+ plasma cell infiltration and fibrosis and demonstrate enhancement on postcontrast imaging series[41] but remains asymptomatic in most cases.[42]

Hepatic involvement

There are several case reports in the literature indicating autoimmune hepatitis in the setting of IgG4-RD,[43,44] but the number of cases are limited and it is not clear if the parenchymal involvement is primary or secondary due to AIP and cholangitis.[45] IgG4-hepathopathy has been described as a general term defining variable liver lesions in patients with IgG4-RD, including pseudotumors, chronic active hepatitis, or extension of IgG4 sclerosing cholangitis to the small portal tracts or bile ducts.[46]

Alimentary tract involvement

Inflammatory bowel disease does not belong to the IgG4-RD spectrum;[47] inflammatory bowel disease is an exclusion for the new IgG4-RD classification criteria (under review for publication). Some have described IgG4-related colitis, but identification of IgG4+ plasma cells in the colon and ileal pouch does not have much diagnostic value because it is a nonspecific finding. IgG4-RD in the alimentary tract can involve glandular tissue and the vascular system resulting in ulcers, polypoid lesions, submucosal masses, or wall thickening. However, gastritis, colitis, and ileitis are not common presentations.[48–50]

Mesenteritis

A few case reports in the literature indicate the presence of characteristic histologic findings of IgG4-RD in sclerosing mesenteritis.[51–53] However, none of the case series[54,55] of sclerosing mesenteritis have a large number of cases with typical systemic features of IgG4-RD, including multiorgan involvement, high serum IgG4 concentrations, tissue IgG4+ plasma cells, and good response to corticosteroid treatment. It can be assumed that if sclerosing mesenteritis is part of a systemic fibrosing process, then it can be considered a manifestation of IgG4-RD, but most isolated cases of sclerosing mesenteritis may be a mimicker of IgG4-RD.

Other Organ Manifestations

Here we discuss the most commonly reported extragastrointestinal organ involvement in IgG4-RD.

Orbits

Ophthalmic presentations of IgG4-RD typically present with periorbital swelling and in some instances frank proptosis secondary to lacrimal gland enlargement as can be seen with dacryoadenitis (**Fig. 1**B).[56] Orbital pseudotumor and extraocular muscle involvement in the form of orbital myositis can cause proptosis with or without lacrimal gland enlargement. Less common reported ophthalmic manifestations have included obstruction of the nasolacrimal duct, scleritis, and compression of peripheral nerves of the orbit.[57,58]

Salivary glands

Both major and minor salivary glands can be affected by IgG4-RD. The most common salivary presentation of IgG4-RD is the painless, firm bilateral enlargement of 2 or more sets of glands (**Fig. 1**C), previously called Mikulicz disease, followed by isolated enlargement of submandibular glands.[59,60] Usually the function of the glands is better preserved compared with primary Sjögren syndrome.

Kidney

The most common form of IgG4-RD in the kidneys is tubulointerstitial nephritis, marked by the histologic findings characteristic of IgG4-RD: lymphoplasmacytic infiltrate with abundance of IgG4+ plasma cells, storiform fibrosis, and moderate tissue eosinophilia.[61] The key difference between renal involvement and other solid organ involvement is the presence of low concentrations of complement, which remains poorly understood but is not believed to be related to IgG4 itself becasue this molecule does not bind complement, and this phenomenon is not largely replicated in most other organs involving IgG4-RD.[62] Clinically, these patients can experience renal dysfunction and even end-stage renal disease if treatment is delayed. Although proteinuria can develop, it is often subnephrotic range proteinuria. Imaging findings will indicate significantly enlarged kidneys and hypodense lesions that are apparent on CT imaging and enhance on postcontrast studies.[63]

Chronic periaortitis and idiopathic retroperitoneal fibrosis

Chronic periaortitis represents a grouping of components, mainly IgG4-related retroperitoneal fibrosis, IgG4-related aortitis, and IgG4-related perianeurysmal fibrosis. Idiopathic retroperitoneal fibrosis is a diagnosis reached after exclusion of secondary causes such as drug exposure, infection, and malignancy.[64] Previously termed Ormond disease, idiopathic retroperitoneal fibrosis is a periaortic or peri-iliac sclerotic disease with encasement of the retroperitoneal structures, particularly the ureters. The most common symptoms can often include flank or abdominal pain, urinary frequency, fatigue, and weight loss. Many cases lead to obstructive nephropathy.[65] Imaging will often reveal a dense soft tissue mass that envelops the abdominal aorta or iliac vessels, with secondary obstructive features leading to unilateral or bilateral hydronephrosis.[66,67]

Lung disease

IgG4-related pulmonary disease presents with a variety of clinical and radiologic manifestations. The most common one is thickening of the bronchovascular bundle, with infiltration of the bronchial wall and blood vessels. Pulmonary nodules, ground-glass opacities, pleural thickening, and interstitial lung disease are among other pulmonary manifestations of IgG4-RD.[68,69] Delayed diagnosis and treatment of IgG4-related interstitial pneumonitis can lead to significant pulmonary fibrosis (see **Fig. 1**C).

DIAGNOSTICS

To date, the most accurate method for diagnosis is clinicopathologic correlation with a detailed clinical history, thorough physical examination complemented by laboratory testing, imaging, and histopathologic examinations. As previously discussed, IgG4-RD usually presents with mass lesions on imaging, mimicking malignancy and making histopathologic examination especially crucial in the diagnosis.

The disease itself does not cause constitutional symptoms or pain, but rather the obstructive nature or cosmetic change in appearance from these tumefactive lesions leads these patients to their physicians. A careful history and physical examination of a patient with painless jaundice may reveal a history of allergies or atopy that has been more recently exacerbated (ie, asthma, eczema, seasonal, or food allergies), a history of recurrent pancreatitis or thyroiditis, or bilateral submandibular gland or lacrimal gland enlargemen, which would give a clue that the presenting painless jaundice is not an isolated phenomenon. Rigorous exclusion of IgG4-RD mimickers is the first and foremost important responsibility of the physicians evaluating patients for this condition.

Laboratory

Serum IgG4 levels

Increased serum IgG4 concentrations were initially a key feature for the diagnosis of IgG4-RD, but it has been found that it is neither necessary nor sufficient for the diagnosis. More recently, a study of a worldwide cohort of patients with IgG4-RD has demonstrated increased IgG4 levels do not confirm the diagnosis and low serum IgG4 levels do not exclude IgG4-RD. Important mimickers of this condition, including pancreatic adenocarcinoma, lymphoma, ANCA-associated vasculitis, and multicentric Castleman disease, can cause increase of serum IgG4 levels, and patients with biopsy-confirmed IgG4-RD can have normal serum IgG4 levels. Carruthers and colleagues[70] showed that the diagnostic utility of serum IgG4 levels is limited because of its poor specificity and low positive predictive value because multiple non-IgG4-RD conditions are associated with modestly increased serum IgG4 levels. In contrast to Carruthers and colleagues,[71] a meta-analysis from China evaluated 22 studies with 6000 white and Asian patients and found a high pooled sensitivity and specificity for serum IgG4. Therefore, the diagnostic yield of an increased serum IgG4 level must be lead to suspicion for IgG4-RD with typical organ involvement in the appropriate setting. A higher serum IgG4 level has higher likelihood of representing IgG4-RD with the observation that a finite number of diseases will cause serum IgG4 concentrations greater than 5 times the upper limit of normal.[72] Patients with IgG4-RD who have involvement of more than 2 organs usually have higher serum IgG4 levels, and it is rare to have normal serum IgG4 with increased load of disease in multiple organ cases. False-negative IgG4 levels due to the prozone phenomenon should be considered in cases with multiorgan involvement and low serum IgG4. Prozone is a phenomenon that can happen during immunoassay for immunoglobulin measurement, a condition in which excess IgG4 occupies only a single binding site on the reagent antibody, preventing immune complex lattice formation, and thereby causing immune complexes to resolubilize and reduce the signal detected by nephelometry or turbidometry.[73]

Monitoring of serum IgG4 concentrations in assessment of disease activity may be useful in only some patients. The serum IgG4 level decreases promptly after treatment with glucocorticoid or B cell depletion in most patients, but many patients do not achieve normal levels while in clinical remission. Disease relapses has been reported to occur in 10% of patients with low serum IgG4 levels.[74] In a prospective trial of rituximab in IgG4-RD, higher baseline increases in serum IgG4, IgE, and blood eosinophil concentrations predicted greater risk of IgG4-RD relapse and shorter time to relapse,[75] making monitoring of these values important.

Other laboratories

Serum IgE levels as well as peripheral eosinophilia have been documented as common features in IgG4-RD in addition to a low titer, positive antinuclear antibody, and rheumatoid factor.[12] Hypocomplementemia has also been found in patients with active disease, although more typically in those patients with renal involvement. Traditional understanding is that IgG4 does not bind complement, which led to further investigation proposing that other IgG subclasses such as IgG1 may have a larger role of complement activation.[76]

Unlike other autoimmune diseases or other infectious, malignant, or inflammatory conditions that would result in increased C-reactive protein level and/or erythrocyte sedimentation rate, these nonspecific markers of inflammation are not typically increased due to IgG4-RD unless another type of inflammation is present at the time of diagnosis as in cases of aortitis or cholangitis.[12] If IgG4-RD is being considered and inflammatory markers are increased, the physician should consider alternative diagnoses in addition to other clinical and/or histologic features to make a diagnosis.

Doorenspleet and colleagues[77] showed a significant role for measurement of dominant IgG4 B cell receptor clones as a biomarker for IgG4-related cholangitis. They initially used next-generation sequencing to show abundance of these clones in both peripheral blood and tissue of patients with IgG4-related cholangitis.[78] More recently, an affordable and practical technique of quantitative polymerase chain reaction to measure the ratio of IgG4/IgG RNA of the same B cell receptors has been proposed and shown to have a sensitivity of 94% and specificity of 99% for diagnosis of IgG4-related cholangitis compared with a sensitivity and specificity of 86% and 73%, respectively, for serum IgG4 alone.[77]

Pathology

Histopathologic evaluation of the affected tissue remains the gold standard for the diagnosis of IgG4-RD because in most cases exclusion of malignancy warrants the biopsy. Usually, needle biopsies and fine-needle aspiration do not provide enough tissue for histologic assessment of IgG4-RD but can be used for exclusion of lymphoma and other malignant conditions.

Characteristic histologic features of IgG4-RD are dense lymphoplasmacytic infiltration, storiform fibrosis (an irregularly cartwheellike fibrotic pattern), and obliterative phlebitis.[79] (**Fig. 2**A) Eosinophilia in mild to moderate amounts and germinal centers

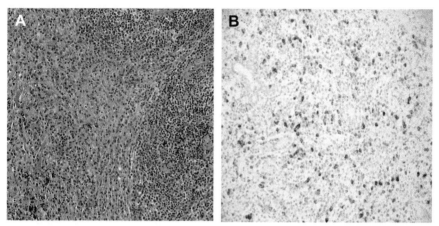

Fig. 2. Pathology of a lacrimal gland in a patient with multisystemic IgG4-RD. (*A*) Low power field view shows significant lymphoplasmacytic infiltration of the submandibular gland with fibrosis (hematoxylin and eosin staining). (*B*) IgG4 immunohistochemical staining of the gland shows marked infiltration of the gland by IgG4+ plasma cells.

are common findings but not necessary for the diagnosis.[80] Prominent neutrophilic infiltration, granuloma, and necrosis are features that would exclude the diagnosis of IgG4-RD and increase the suspicion for infections, sarcoidosis, or granulomatosis with polyangiitis. In addition to the histology, presence of IgG4+ plasma cells infiltrating the tissue is necessary (**Fig. 2**B). Performance of immunohistochemistry on biopsy samples is essential for the diagnosis of IgG4-RD to evaluate the number of IgG4+ plasma cells and the IgG4/IgG ratio.[80,81] Relying solely on the number of IgG4+ plasma cells can be dangerous because many mimickers of IgG4-RD can have a high number of IgG4 plasma cells. Although histology and immunohistochemistry features are the key for diagnosis, similar findings in certain tissues in the absence of typical organ involvement may be considered nonspecific. Skin, lymph node, thyroid, and nasal sinus cavities are among the sites that can show IgG4+ plasma cells in the setting of fibroinflammation without specificity.

TREATMENT

To date there have been no randomized controlled studies on the treatment of IgG4-RD; therefore, the best evidence-based therapy for this condition is not known. Observational studies and international consensus statements regarding management and treatment considered most of the evidence for the efficacy of certain therapies for induction of remission and lowering relapse rates.[82,83]

Glucocorticoid Treatment

Glucocorticoids are the mainstay of therapy for this disease entity, so much so, that response to such therapy has been part of the diagnostic criteria for type 1 AIP.[32] In most studies to date, glucocorticoids are used for induction therapy for IgG4-RD and in certain instances, low doses of glucocorticoid equivalent to prednisone 5 to 7.5 mg daily for maintenance therapy.

The international consensus guidelines on the management of IgG4-RD recommends 2 to 4 weeks of induction therapy with a prednisone equivalent of 30 or 0.6 mg/kg. This dose is then tapered over a period of 8 to 12 weeks, during which the disease is frequently documented to relapse.[82,84] The same induction therapy is used again with the original higher doses of glucocorticoids. Physicians will often choose to start a steroid-sparing agent or regimen after the first relapse although if some patients are able to achieve disease activity remission, maintenance therapy may be continued with low-dose glucocorticoids.

Steroid-Sparing Agents

There is a limited amount of evidence for use of steroid-sparing agents in IgG4-RD, making the decision for a treatment strategy difficult for clinicians. A systematic review from 2016 by Brito-Zeron and colleagues[83] found that azathioprine was used in 85% of cases when a steroid-sparing agent was used, followed in decreasing frequency by mycophenolate mofetil, methotrexate, tacrolimus, leflunomide, and cyclophospha-mide. The same systematic review reported relapse rates on low doses of azathioprine (ie, 50 mg daily) and mycophenolate (ie, 1 g daily) and further reported decreased relapse rates on escalated doses of each. Further review of the corresponding series revealed that these dose escalations were done in conjunction with glucocorticoids, which as stated above are considered to be the mainstay of therapy, therefore con-founding the ability to assess efficacy of these steroid-sparing agents.

To date, there has not been a head to head comparison of specific conventional steroid-sparing agents. Studies on AIP in particular indicate use of azathioprine by gastroenterologists as the steroid-sparing agent of choice.[85]

Rituximab has been shown to be effective in the treatment of patients with IgG4-RD in many case series and a prospective open label study of 30 patients.[14,86] Thus, rit-uximab is now considered the first steroid-sparing agent in clinical practice for IgG4-RD, at least in countries where this medication is available.[87]

Other biologics, including bortezomib, infliximab, and abatacept, have been re-ported to be effective in this condition but data are limited to single case reports.[88–90]

Stents

As previously described, IgG4-RD is a fibroinflammatory condition wherein delays in prompt treatment can lead to significant fibrosis and damage that is refractory to both glucocorticoids and immunosuppressive therapy. This fibrosis leads to mechan-ical obstruction and organ dysfunction, which can be alleviated mechanically with stents.

For example, in the setting of obstructive jaundice secondary to IgG4-related chol-angitis, endoscopic placement of metal or plastic stents plays a role for relieving obstruction from biliary strictures.[91] This idea is replicated in IgG4-related retroperito-neal fibrosis with case reports documenting a benefit of ureteral stenting in the setting of ureteral obstruction and resultant hydronephrosis.[92,93]

SUMMARY

IgG4-RD is an under-recognized fibroinflammatory condition marked by tumefactive lesions that mimic malignancy, infectious disorders, or other inflammatory conditions such as granulomatous polyangiitis. Lesions in multiple organ systems can be syn-chronous at the time of diagnosis or metachronous over the patient's lifetime. Delays in diagnosis can lead to dysfunction of solid organs or progressive fibrosis that can cause irreversible damage such as cirrhosis, renal failure, aneurysms of the thoracic or abdominal aorta, or loss of vision. Many patients will undergo invasive procedures for biopsy or resection of lesions to exclude other conditions but will not have specific evaluation for IgG4-RD. Definitive diagnosis requires a histopathologic evaluation, generally by biopsy in addition to insightful correlation with the patient's history and physical examination as well as radiology and laboratory findings.

Although increased serum IgG4 concentrations and increasing recognition of IgG4-positive plasma cells in tissue are among the diagnostic criteria, there is variability in the accuracy of assays and values of serum IgG4 in biopsy-proven diagnoses—to the point where many researchers and clinicians disregard the use of serum IgG4 when making or validating a diagnosis.

One of the hallmarks of this condition is its response to glucocorticoid therapy, generally dramatic in nature, leading to exclusion of a diagnosis if there is no response to steroid. Although there are some patients who will respond and have complete remission after a short period of use of glucocorticoids, there are still others who will require an efficacious steroid-sparing agent for maintenance therapy. This need is further highlighted by the known side effect profile of long-term glucocorticoid use and even more so in those patients with IgG4-related pancreatic insufficiency and resultant diabetes. In our review, we have highlighted currently available therapies that are used globally by clinicians treating IgG4-RD.

REFERENCES

1. Kawaguchi K, Koike M, Tsuruta K, et al. Lymphoplasmacytic sclerosing pancreatitis with cholangitis: a variant of primary sclerosing cholangitis extensively involving pancreas. Hum Pathol 1991;22(4):387–95.
2. Yoshida K, Toki F, Takeuchi T, et al. Chronic pancreatitis caused by an autoimmune abnormality. Proposal of the concept of autoimmune pancreatitis. Dig Dis Sci 1995;40(7):1561–8.
3. Hamano H, Kawa S, Horiuchi A, et al. High serum IgG4 concentrations in patients with sclerosing pancreatitis. N Engl J Med 2001;344(10):732–8.
4. Kamisawa T, Okamoto A. Autoimmune pancreatitis: proposal of IgG4-related sclerosing disease. J Gastroenterol 2006;41(7):613–25.
5. Stone JH, Khosroshahi A, Deshpande V, et al. Recommendations for the nomenclature of IgG4-related disease and its individual organ system manifestations. Arthritis Rheum 2012;64(10):3061–7.
6. Kamisawa T, Zen Y, Pillai S, et al. IgG4-related disease. Lancet 2015;385(9976): 1460–71.
7. Wallace ZS, Stone JH. An update on IgG4-related disease. Curr Opin Rheumatol 2015;27(1):83–90.
8. Culver EL, Sadler R, Simpson D, et al. Elevated serum IgG4 levels in diagnosis, treatment response, organ involvement, and relapse in a prospective IgG4-related disease UK cohort. Am J Gastroenterol 2016;111(5):733–43.
9. Brito-Zeron P, Ramos-Casals M, Bosch X, et al. The clinical spectrum of IgG4-related disease. Autoimmun Rev 2014;13(12):1203–10.
10. Kanno A, Masamune A, Okazaki K, et al. Nationwide epidemiological survey of autoimmune pancreatitis in Japan in 2011. Pancreas 2015;44(4):535–9.
11. Inoue D, Yoshida K, Yoneda N, et al. IgG4-related disease: dataset of 235 consecutive patients. Medicine (Baltimore) 2015;94(15):e680.
12. Wallace ZS, Deshpande V, Mattoo H, et al. IgG4-related disease: clinical and laboratory features in one hundred twenty-five patients. Arthritis Rheumatol 2015; 67(9):2466–75.
13. Zen Y, Nakanuma Y. IgG4-related disease: a cross-sectional study of 114 cases. Am J Surg Pathol 2010;34(12):1812–9.

14. Carruthers MN, Topazian MD, Khosroshahi A, et al. Rituximab for IgG4-related disease: a prospective, open-label trial. Ann Rheum Dis 2015;74(6):1171–7.
15. Khosroshahi A, Carruthers MN, Deshpande V, et al. Rituximab for the treatment of IgG4-related disease: lessons from 10 consecutive patients. Medicine (Baltimore) 2012;91(1):57–66.
16. Ebbo M, Grados A, Samson M, et al. Long-term efficacy and safety of rituximab in IgG4-related disease: data from a French nationwide study of thirty-three patients. PLoS One 2017;12(9):e0183844.
17. Della-Torre E, Lanzillotta M, Doglioni C. Immunology of IgG4-related disease. Clin Exp Immunol 2015;181(2):191–206.
18. Odendahl M, Jacobi A, Hansen A, et al. Disturbed peripheral B lymphocyte homeostasis in systemic lupus erythematosus. J Immunol 2000;165(10):5970–9.
19. Wallace ZS, Mattoo H, Carruthers M, et al. Plasmablasts as a biomarker for IgG4-related disease, independent of serum IgG4 concentrations. Ann Rheum Dis 2015;74(1):190–5.
20. de Buy Wenniger LJ, Culver EL, Beuers U. Exposure to occupational antigens might predispose to IgG4-related disease. Hepatology 2014;60(4):1453–4.
21. Zen Y, Fujii T, Harada K, et al. Th2 and regulatory immune reactions are increased in immunoglobin G4-related sclerosing pancreatitis and cholangitis. Hepatology 2007;45(6):1538–46.
22. Vinuesa CG, Tangye SG, Moser B, et al. Follicular B helper T cells in antibody responses and autoimmunity. Nat Rev Immunol 2005;5(11):853–65.
23. Akiyama M, Suzuki K, Yasuoka H, et al. Follicular helper T cells in the pathogenesis of IgG4-related disease. Rheumatology (Oxford) 2018;57(2):236–45.
24. Akiyama M, Yasuoka H, Yamaoka K, et al. Enhanced IgG4 production by follicular helper 2 T cells and the involvement of follicular helper 1 T cells in the pathogenesis of IgG4-related disease. Arthritis Res Ther 2016;18:167.
25. Miyabe K, Zen Y, Cornell LD, et al. Gastrointestinal and extra-intestinal manifestations of immunoglobulin G4-related disease. Gastroenterology 2018;155(4):990–1003.e1.
26. Lin W, Lu S, Chen H, et al. Clinical characteristics of immunoglobulin G4-related disease: a prospective study of 118 Chinese patients. Rheumatology (Oxford) 2015;54(11):1982–90.
27. Sekiguchi H, Horie R, Kanai M, et al. IgG4-related disease: retrospective analysis of one hundred sixty-six patients. Arthritis Rheumatol 2016;68(9):2290–9.
28. Chari ST, Smyrk TC, Levy MJ, et al. Diagnosis of autoimmune pancreatitis: the mayo clinic experience. Clin Gastroenterol Hepatol 2006;4(8):1010–6 [quiz: 1934].
29. Nagpal SJS, Sharma A, Chari ST. Autoimmune pancreatitis. Am J Gastroenterol 2018;113(9):1301.
30. Deshpande V, Gupta R, Sainani N, et al. Subclassification of autoimmune pancreatitis: a histologic classification with clinical significance. Am J Surg Pathol 2011;35(1):26–35.
31. Zamboni G, Luttges J, Capelli P, et al. Histopathological features of diagnostic and clinical relevance in autoimmune pancreatitis: a study on 53 resection specimens and 9 biopsy specimens. Virchows Arch 2004;445(6):552–63.
32. Shimosegawa T, Chari ST, Frulloni L, et al. International consensus diagnostic criteria for autoimmune pancreatitis: guidelines of the International Association of Pancreatology. Pancreas 2011;40(3):352–8.
33. Nakazawa T, Notohara K, Tazuma S, et al. The 2016 diagnostic criteria for primary sclerosing cholangitis. J Gastroenterol 2017;52(7):838–44.

34. Tang CSW, Sivarasan N, Griffin N. Abdominal manifestations of IgG4-related disease: a pictorial review. Insights Imaging 2018;9(4):437–48.

35. Vlachou PA, Khalili K, Jang HJ, et al. IgG4-related sclerosing disease: autoimmune pancreatitis and extrapancreatic manifestations. Radiographics 2011; 31(5):1379–402.

36. Kalaitzakis E, Levy M, Kamisawa T, et al. Endoscopic retrograde cholangiography does not reliably distinguish IgG4-associated cholangitis from primary sclerosing cholangitis or cholangiocarcinoma. Clin Gastroenterol Hepatol 2011; 9(9):800–3.e2.

37. Nakazawa T, Ohara H, Sano H, et al. Cholangiography can discriminate sclerosing cholangitis with autoimmune pancreatitis from primary sclerosing cholangitis. Gastrointest Endosc 2004;60(6):937–44.

38. Itoi T, Kamisawa T, Igarashi Y, et al. The role of peroral video cholangioscopy in patients with IgG4-related sclerosing cholangitis. J Gastroenterol 2013;48(4): 504–14.

39. Nakazawa T, Ando T, Hayashi K, et al. Diagnostic procedures for IgG4-related sclerosing cholangitis. J Hepatobiliary Pancreat Sci 2011;18(2):127–36.

40. Kojima E, Kimura K, Noda Y, et al. Autoimmune pancreatitis and multiple bile duct strictures treated effectively with steroid. J Gastroenterol 2003;38(6):603–7.

41. Kamisawa T, Egawa N, Nakajima H, et al. Extrapancreatic lesions in autoimmune pancreatitis. J Clin Gastroenterol 2005;39(10):904–7.

42. Kamisawa T, Takuma K, Egawa N, et al. Autoimmune pancreatitis and IgG4-related sclerosing disease. Nat Rev Gastroenterol Hepatol 2010;7(7):401–9.

43. Umemura T, Zen Y, Hamano H, et al. IgG4 associated autoimmune hepatitis: a differential diagnosis for classical autoimmune hepatitis. Gut 2007;56(10): 1471–2.

44. Nakanuma Y, Ishizu Y, Zen Y, et al. Histopathology of IgG4-related autoimmune hepatitis and IgG4-related hepatopathy in IgG4-related disease. Semin Liver Dis 2016;36(3):229–41.

45. Naitoh I, Zen Y, Nakazawa T, et al. Small bile duct involvement in IgG4-related sclerosing cholangitis: liver biopsy and cholangiography correlation. J Gastroenterol 2011;46(2):269–76.

46. Hirano K, Shiratori Y, Komatsu Y, et al. Involvement of the biliary system in autoimmune pancreatitis: a follow-up study. Clin Gastroenterol Hepatol 2003;1(6): 453–64.

47. Lew M, Deshpande V. IgG4-related disorders of the gastrointestinal tract. Surg Pathol Clin 2013;6(3):497–521.

48. Cheong HR, Lee BE, Song GA, et al. Immunoglobulin G4-related inflammatory pseudotumor presenting as a solitary mass in the stomach. Clin Endosc 2016; 49(2):197–201.

49. Baez JC, Hamilton MJ, Bellizzi A, et al. Gastric involvement in autoimmune pancreatitis: MDCT and histopathologic features. JOP 2010;11(6):610–3.

50. Kawano H, Ishii A, Kimura T, et al. IgG4-related disease manifesting the gastric wall thickening. Pathol Int 2016;66(1):23–8.

51. Mori E, Kamisawa T, Tabata T, et al. A case of IgG4-related mesenteritis. Clin J Gastroenterol 2015;8(6):400–5.

52. Chen TS, Montgomery EA. Are tumefactive lesions classified as sclerosing mesenteritis a subset of IgG4-related sclerosing disorders? J Clin Pathol 2008;61(10): 1093–7.

53. Minato H, Shimizu J, Arano Y, et al. IgG4-related sclerosing mesenteritis: a rare mesenteric disease of unknown etiology. Pathol Int 2012;62(4):281–6.

54. Emory TS, Monihan JM, Carr NJ, et al. Sclerosing mesenteritis, mesenteric panniculitis and mesenteric lipodystrophy: a single entity? Am J Surg Pathol 1997; 21(4):392–8.
55. Akram S, Pardi DS, Schaffner JA, et al. Sclerosing mesenteritis: clinical features, treatment, and outcome in ninety-two patients. Clin Gastroenterol Hepatol 2007; 5(5):589–96 [quiz: 523–4].
56. Wallace ZS, Deshpande V, Stone JH. Ophthalmic manifestations of IgG4-related disease: single-center experience and literature review. Semin Arthritis Rheum 2014;43(6):806–17.
57. Wallace ZS, Khosroshahi A, Jakobiec FA, et al. IgG4-related systemic disease as a cause of "idiopathic" orbital inflammation, including orbital myositis, and trigeminal nerve involvement. Surv Ophthalmol 2012;57(1):26–33.
58. Ohno K, Sato Y, Ohshima K, et al. IgG4-related disease involving the sclera. Mod Rheumatol 2014;24(1):195–8.
59. Himi T, Takano K, Yamamoto M, et al. A novel concept of Mikulicz's disease as IgG4-related disease. Auris Nasus Larynx 2012;39(1):9–17.
60. Yamamoto M, Takahashi H, Sugai S, et al. Clinical and pathological characteristics of Mikulicz's disease (IgG4-related plasmacytic exocrinopathy). Autoimmun Rev 2005;4(4):195–200.
61. Saeki T, Nishi S, Imai N, et al. Clinicopathological characteristics of patients with IgG4-related tubulointerstitial nephritis. Kidney Int 2010;78(10):1016–23.
62. Saeki T, Ito T, Yamazaki H, et al. Hypocomplementemia of unknown etiology: an opportunity to find cases of IgG4-positive multi-organ lymphoproliferative syndrome. Rheumatol Int 2009;30(1):99–103.
63. Saeki T, Kawano M, Mizushima I, et al. The clinical course of patients with IgG4-related kidney disease. Kidney Int 2013;84(4):826–33.
64. Vaglio A, Palmisano A, Corradi D, et al. Retroperitoneal fibrosis: evolving concepts. Rheum Dis Clin North Am 2007;33(4):803–17, vi-vii.
65. van Bommel EF, Jansen I, Hendriksz TR, et al. Idiopathic retroperitoneal fibrosis: prospective evaluation of incidence and clinicoradiologic presentation. Medicine (Baltimore) 2009;88(4):193–201.
66. Corradi D, Maestri R, Palmisano A, et al. Idiopathic retroperitoneal fibrosis: clinicopathologic features and differential diagnosis. Kidney Int 2007;72(6):742–53.
67. Scheel PJ Jr, Feeley N. Retroperitoneal fibrosis: the clinical, laboratory, and radiographic presentation. Medicine (Baltimore) 2009;88(4):202–7.
68. Zen Y, Inoue D, Kitao A, et al. IgG4-related lung and pleural disease: a clinicopathologic study of 21 cases. Am J Surg Pathol 2009;33(12):1886–93.
69. Inoue D, Zen Y, Abo H, et al. Immunoglobulin G4-related lung disease: CT findings with pathologic correlations. Radiology 2009;251(1):260–70.
70. Carruthers MN, Khosroshahi A, Augustin T, et al. The diagnostic utility of serum IgG4 concentrations in IgG4-related disease. Ann Rheum Dis 2015;74(1):14–8.
71. Xu WL, Ling YC, Wang ZK, et al. Diagnostic performance of serum IgG4 level for IgG4-related disease: a meta-analysis. Sci Rep 2016;6:32035.
72. Boonstra K, Culver EL, de Buy Wenniger LM, et al. Serum immunoglobulin G4 and immunoglobulin G1 for distinguishing immunoglobulin G4-associated cholangitis from primary sclerosing cholangitis. Hepatology 2014;59(5):1954–63.
73. Khosroshahi A, Cheryk LA, Carruthers MN, et al. Brief report: spuriously low serum IgG4 concentrations caused by the prozone phenomenon in patients with IgG4-related disease. Arthritis Rheumatol 2014;66(1):213–7.
74. Kamisawa T, Shimosegawa T, Okazaki K, et al. Standard steroid treatment for autoimmune pancreatitis. Gut 2009;58(11):1504–7.

75. Wallace ZS, Mattoo H, Mahajan VS, et al. Predictors of disease relapse in IgG4-related disease following rituximab. Rheumatology (Oxford) 2016;55(6):1000–8.
76. Kawa S. The immunobiology of immunoglobulin G4 and complement activation pathways in IgG4-related disease. Curr Top Microbiol Immunol 2017;401:61–73.
77. Doorenspleet ME, Hubers LM, Culver EL, et al. Immunoglobulin G4(+) B-cell receptor clones distinguish immunoglobulin G 4-related disease from primary sclerosing cholangitis and biliary/pancreatic malignancies. Hepatology 2016;64(2): 501–7.
78. Maillette de Buy Wenniger LJ, Doorenspleet ME, Klarenbeek PL, et al. Immunoglobulin G4+ clones identified by next-generation sequencing dominate the B cell receptor repertoire in immunoglobulin G4 associated cholangitis. Hepatology 2013;57(6):2390–8.
79. Ghably JG, Borthwick T, O'Neil TJ, et al. IgG4-related disease: a primer on diagnosis and management. Ann Allergy Asthma Immunol 2015;114(6):447–54.
80. Bateman AC, Culver EL. IgG4-related disease – experience of 100 consecutive cases from a specialist centre. Histopathology 2017;70(5):798–813.
81. Masaki Y, Kurose N, Yamamoto M, et al. Cutoff values of serum IgG4 and histopathological IgG4+ plasma cells for diagnosis of patients with IgG4-related disease. Int J Rheumatol 2012;2012:580814.
82. Khosroshahi A, Wallace ZS, Crowe JL, et al. International consensus guidance statement on the management and treatment of IgG4-related disease. Arthritis Rheumatol 2015;67(7):1688–99.
83. Brito-Zeron P, Kostov B, Bosch X, et al. Therapeutic approach to IgG4-related disease: a systematic review. Medicine (Baltimore) 2016;95(26):e4002.
84. Hart PA, Topazian MD, Witzig TE, et al. Treatment of relapsing autoimmune pancreatitis with immunomodulators and rituximab: the Mayo Clinic experience. Gut 2013;62(11):1607–15.
85. Hart PA, Kamisawa T, Brugge WR, et al. Long-term outcomes of autoimmune pancreatitis: a multicentre, international analysis. Gut 2013;62(12):1771–6.
86. Khosroshahi A, Bloch DB, Deshpande V, et al. Rituximab therapy leads to rapid decline of serum IgG4 levels and prompt clinical improvement in IgG4-related systemic disease. Arthritis Rheum 2010;62(6):1755–62.
87. Yamamoto M, Awakawa T, Takahashi H. Is rituximab effective for IgG4-related disease in the long term? Experience of cases treated with rituximab for 4 years. Ann Rheum Dis 2015;74(8):e46.
88. Khan ML, Colby TV, Viggiano RW, et al. Treatment with bortezomib of a patient having hyper IgG4 disease. Clin Lymphoma Myeloma Leuk 2010;10(3):217–9.
89. Balaskas K, de Leval L, La Corte R, et al. Infliximab therapy for a severe case of IgG4-related ocular adnexal disorder recalcitrant to corticosteroid treatment. Ocul Immunol Inflamm 2012;20(6):478–80.
90. Yamamoto M, Takahashi H, Takano K, et al. Efficacy of abatacept for IgG4-related disease over 8 months. Ann Rheum Dis 2016;75(8):1576–8.
91. Mahajan A, Ho H, Sauer B, et al. Temporary placement of fully covered self-expandable metal stents in benign biliary strictures: midterm evaluation (with video). Gastrointest Endosc 2009;70(2):303–9.
92. Maeta S, Munemura C, Ishida C, et al. Case report; acute renal failure due to IgG4-related retroperitoneal fibrosis. Nihon Naika Gakkai Zasshi 2012;101(4): 1079–81 [in Japanese].
93. Zhang W, Xue F, Wang C, et al. Clinical features and prognostic factors of ten patients with renal failure caused by IgG4-related retroperitoneal fibrosis. Oncotarget 2018;9(2):2858–65.

Serologic Diagnosis of Celiac Disease: New Biomarkers

Aaron Lerner, MD, MHA[a,b,*], Ajay Ramesh, PhD[b],
Torsten Matthias, PhD[b]

KEYWORDS

- Celiac disease • Diagnosis • Serologic marker
- Neo-epitope tissue transglutaminase • Antibody

KEY POINTS

- Celiac disease is a multi-face disease and most of the affected persons are a/hyposymptomatic and underdiagnosed.
- With improvements, serologic markers became very important for screening and diagnosing celiac disease.
- Multiple serologic biomarkers exist in celiac disease, but IgA anti-endomysial antibodies (AEA), IgA-tTg, and neo-epitope tTg check are the most reliable ones.
- In the setting of IgA-deficient patients with celiac disease, IgA and IgG isotype serologic testing should be considered.

INTRODUCTION

A decade ago, the letters "GF" in the supermarket or on a restaurant menu were likely unknown and confused many people. Now, a gluten-free lifestyle has increasingly become the most popular diet trend in the United States. According to a 2015 Gallup poll and a report by Moore[1] 20% to 30% of the US population reduces or eliminates gluten consumption, the main protein of wheat. Kim and colleagues[2] have found that women are more likely than men to avoid gluten, and the diet is most popular among 20- to 39-year-olds.

Because the diagnosis of CD relies on symptoms, small intestine pathology, and associated serology, the western trend to withdraw gluten may have consequences for the diagnostic reliability of serology because tTG antibody may wane on a

No grant support. T. Matthias is the head and owner of the AESKU group. AESKU.Diagnostics is producing and selling the neo-epitope tTg antibody.
[a] B. Rappaport School of Medicine, Technion-Israel Institute of Technology, Haifa, Israel;
[b] AESKU.KIPP Institute, Mikroforum Ring 2, Wendelsheim 55234, Germany
* Corresponding author. AESKU.KIPP Institute, Mikroforum Ring 2, Wendelsheim 55234, Germany.
E-mail address: aaronlerner1948@gmail.com

gluten-free diet.[3] CD and CD incidence is only 1%, albeit rates are reportedly increasing constantly.[4,5]

Celiac Disease

Celiac disease is an autoimmune, mainly enteric, disease affecting multiple nongastrointestinal organs and peripheral tissues. Precipitated in genetically predisposed individuals by the ingestion of prolamins, a major class of storage proteins found in wheat, rye, barley, and less in oat, but which are mainly represented by gluten that comprise 80% of wheat proteins. Being an autoimmune disease, it is almost by definition, genetically determined, and environmentally induced. The genetic predisposition is related to human leukocyte antigen DQ2 and DQ8 haplotypes, but more than 50 associated genes have been described.[6] CD affects 1.0% to 1.5% of the population worldwide, with wide differences in European countries.[4,5] Its epidemiology and clinical presentation are constantly changing. It has been shown that the classic intestinal clinical picture of malnutrition, chronic diarrhea, and nutritional deficiencies are decreasing and extraintestinal presentations are emerging. Skin, endocrine, skeletal, hepatic, hematologic, thrombophilic, gynecologic, fertility, dental, cutaneous, neurologic, and behavioral abnormalities are often described.[7,8] Despite being a silent or slowly developing chronic condition, it can present acutely[9] and even as obesity or constipation.[10,11] For the last decades, we are witnessing an epidemiologic shift toward a more advanced patient age, and increased prevalence of latent, hyposymptomatic, or asymptomatic cases.[6–9]

Why Celiac Disease Should be Diagnosed as Early as Possible?

Under diagnosis and long diagnostic delay have substantial implications, in terms of morbidity, mortality, and economic burden. Gluten-free diet was shown to reduce complications, realize potential growth and weight parameters, improve pregnancy outcome, enhance bone density, decrease co-occurrence of several autoimmune conditions, shorten needless suffering, prevent malignancies, and overall improve life quality and expectancy. The title "Pediatric celiac disease: early diagnosis for better lifelong health" summarizes and reinforces the early diagnosis of the disease.[12]

CELIAC DISEASE DIAGNOSTIC SEROLOGIC MARKERS

Before detailing the plethora of serologic markers, respect should be given to the history and discoverers of those antibodies. **Table 1** depicts the history of CD antibodies.

The case-finding strategy of CD is debatable, ranging between prioritizing serologic biomarkers to duodenal biopsies and various combinations between the two.[3,25,26] In

Table 1
The history of the serologic markers in celiac disease

Antibody	Year of Discovery	References
Anti-gliadin	1983	13,14
Anti-endomysial	1983	15,16
Anti-tissue transglutaminase	1997	17,18
Anti-deamidated gliadin peptide	2001	19,20
Anti-neo-epitope tTg	2010	21,22
Anti-neo-epitope mTg	2016	23,24

Abbreviations: mTg, microbial transglutaminase; tTg, tissue transglutaminase.

fact, the diagnostic strategies are different in various countries and continents and are age dependent, as was extensively and most recently summarized by Turner.[3] The debate on the gold standard for pediatric and adult CD diagnosis is heated and ongoing. It is not only the race for the best serologic marker, but also the diagnostic reliability of intestinal pathology. Intestinal biopsy was for decades the ultimate standard, but because of incorrect interpretation, disuniformity in grading gut histology using revised Marsh criteria, lack of agreement on the cut-off number of intraepithelial lymphocytes (a hallmark of CD intestinal injury), and the fact that histologic features of CD are not specific, all raise a question mark on the pathologic standard.[27–30] Parallel to the progress in CD serologic reliability, the antibodies came to occupy a higher role in the CD workup.[31] This is clearly reflected in the most recent ESPGHAN criteria, published in 2012.[32] Noteworthy, none of the other pediatric or adult gastroenterology societies adopted those criteria. In brief, according to the ESPGHAN criteria, a symptomatic child with an IgA-tTg titer > x10 upper limit of normal, with a positive anti-endomysial antibody (AEA) having HLA-DQ2/8, is exempt from a diagnostic endoscopy. It should be mentioned that multiple publications encourage the reliability, accuracy, and applicability of those criteria.[33–36] Conversely, many argue against them, calling for revised criteria and adopting duodenal histology as the gold standard.[3,37–43] Many express the need to ease the diagnosis of CD,[44] or modify the diagnostic approach for certain clinical circumstances.[45] Taken together, CD represents a diagnostic challenge and the jury has not completed deliberations.[46] Despite the open challenges, CD-associated antibodies can be graded for diagnostic performance and limitation based on current knowledge.

The Classic Serologic Markers of Celiac Disease

Celiac disease serology can be divided chronologically starting with the classic older markers established before 2010 (anti-gliadin antibodies [AGA], AEA, deamidated gliadin peptide [DGP] and tTg) then considering the more recent ones that appeared on the market since 2010, namely anti-neo-epitope tTg (see **Table 1**). Here might be the correct place to stress that, generally, combined antibodies perform better than a single one.[31,47] The following paragraphs describe the strengths and the drawbacks of those CD biomarkers.

Anti-gliadin antibodies was the first serologic test to inform the need for intestinal, gold standard, diagnostic sampling. It is directed against a nutritional protein, namely, gliadin or gluten and contrary to the other markers, gliaden tests for is not an autoantibody. The accuracy of the antibodies against native gliadin is limited. Their sensitivity and specificity are generally less than 90% with positive predicted values much less than 50%.[14,48] They appear in normal controls, increase with age, are genetically determined, are gluten dependent, and are shared between multiple gastrointestinal and autoimmune diseases.[14,49]

Because of their low performance and the availability of much better serologic markers, AGA IgA and IgG antibodies fell out of favor and were replaced with the better performing DGP antibodies.[50]

Anti-endomysium antibodies belong primarily to the IgA class and is directed against the intermyofibril substance of smooth muscle, as checked on monkey esophagus endomysium by indirect immunofluorescent assay.[15,16,51] Anti-endomysium antibodies performs better in children, reaching specificity of greater than 95% but their sensitivity is lower than 90%. The diagnostic reliability is lower in children less than 2 years of age, and in the elderly, and in the face of milder intestinal injury.[31,50] The disadvantages are their higher cost and being labor-intensive to perform and nonobjective with a significant interobserver and intersite variability. Despite those pitfalls, they were included on the revised diagnostic flow chart of ESPGHAN 2012.[32] Nowadays, they are less widely performed and were replaced by more reliable, reproducible, and objective ones.

IgA to tissue transglutaminase is the most used and studied marker in CD and is primarily recommended by ESPGHAN.[32] It is directed against the ubiquitous enzyme tTg, the identified autoantigen of CD.[17,18,52–54] It is a reliable, inexpensive, and reproducible test, performed by enzyme-linked immunosorbent assay. IgA-tTg sensitivity and specificity are generally considered greater than 90–95%, but have a wide range between 74% and 100% depending on performing laboratory and kit used.[31] Most frequently, human recombinant tTg is used as an antigen in the bottom of the microtiter well. Despite its frequent use, the medical and the laboratory teams should be aware regarding its many false-positive and false-negative characteristics.[55,56] **Table 2** summarizes the false positivity and negativity of the IgA-tTg, as adapted from references.[55–57] Despite these shortcomings, IgA-tTg antibodies reflect the CD intestinal damage and can predict the enteric pathology.[22,32,57,58]

Taken together, the sensitivity of tTg autoantibodies is slightly higher in comparison with the AEA, while the specificity of AEA is slightly higher than that of tTg.[59] IgA-tTg autoantibodies are currently the most evaluated and widely accepted serologic marker of CD.

Deamidated gliadin peptide antigen is the intestinal form of gliadin deamidated by tTg, thus improving its binding to the antigen-presenting cell's HLA groove, is better presented to the lamina propria CD4$^+$ T cells[6,52] and therefore starts the inflammatory cascade. IgA-DGP antibodies have a specificity of greater than 90% and sensitivity of greater than 80% in children, and less in adults.[31] The combined IgA + IgG isotypes perform much better. It has a low positive predicted value[60,61] and may not have the

Table 2 Pitfalls in tTg autoantibody testing	
False-Positive tTg	**False-Negative tTg**
In face of Marsh 1, degree of intestinal injury	Complete IgA deficiency
Autoimmune diseases: IBD, primary biliary cirrhosis, Goodpasture syndrome, granulomatosis with polyangiitis (Wegener type), rheumatoid arthritis, SLE, systemic sclerosis, type 1 diabetes, pemphigus, and psoriasis	Refractory CD
Nonautoimmune disease: connective tissue diseases, nonautoimmune cirrhosis, linear IgA dermatosis, herpes gestationis, vasculitis	Small intestinal bacterial overgrowth
Increased IgM rheumatic factor	Age dependency, especially in the elderly
In face of positive anti-endomysial antibody	In face of anti-tTg subepithelial deposits
Transient, fluctuating positivity	During gluten-free diet
Childhood cerebral palsy	Some nonatrophic patients with CD
Infectious febrile diseases	Transient, fluctuating negativity
End-stage heart failure	Genetic risk
Down syndrome	Viral infections
Neoplastic conditions	Immune deficiency/suppression
Following Epstein-Barr virus infection	

Abbreviations: IBD, inflammatory bowel disease; SLE, systemic lupus erythematosus.

diagnostic value required as an additional screening test to anti-tTg antibodies for identifying patients with CD.[62] Anti-DGP increases neither the sensitivity nor the specificity of AEA and anti-tTg antibodies.[63] In addition, IgA-DGP show inferior diagnostic accuracy when compared with AEA and IgA-tTg.[64] Despite praising anti-IgG-DGP, as the best CD diagnostic marker for less than 2 years age,[65] most probably, it is the combination of IgA-tTg and IgG-DGP that outperforms the single antibodies.[66] Finally, a meta-analysis of all available publications on DGPs, published in 2010, showed that the tTg determinations still outperform DGP-based assays. The authors stressed that most of the screened publications are biased and thus may result in false-positive sensitivity values.[67]

The New Serologic Markers of Celiac Disease

Before reviewing the new generation of CD diagnostic antibodies, the concept of neo-epitope complex formation by posttranslational modification of naive proteins should be discussed.

The concept of posttranslationally modified proteins: transglutaminases as modifiers of gluten

The role of enzymatic posttranslational modification of nutrients and non-nutritional proteins in the gut lumen, in autoimmunity induction, was reviewed recently.[68,69] Being rich in glutamine, gluten is an ideal substrate for the tranglutaminase family to deamidate or transamidate (crosslink to an acyl acceptor).[70] Because tTg is the autoantigen in CD and since microbial transglutaminase (mTg) imitates functionally tTg, both are modifiers of gluten.[68] Interestingly, mTg is heavily used in the processed food industries, including bakeries[71] and is also secreted by the gut microbiota[68,69]; both enzymes, tTg and mTg, modify gluten in the gut lumen and in the enteric mucosa, respectively. The following is the appropriate place to explain the notion of the neo-epitope formation and its immunogenic capacity.

Neo-epitope tissue/microbial transglutaminase antibodies

Matthias and colleagues[21,72] were the first to suggest that autoantibodies against the complex, created by the endogenous tTg crosslinking gliadin, occur in patients with CD. This posttranslational modification creates a significant change in the 3D structure of the complex, exposing neo-epitopes that are presented to the CD mucosal immune system. Following the docking of gliadin on the active site of the enzyme, naive gliadin peptides are transformed, losing their tolerogenic behavior, acquire immunogenicity and induce autoantibodies targeting epitopes designated "neo-epitope." The complex formation, their uptake and processing by the antigen-presenting cells support the epitope spreading from neo-epitopes to gliadin peptides and tTg.[72–76]

A parallel pathway is created when the exogenous mTg is crosslinking gluten or gliadin peptides, as extensively reported recently.[24,58,70]

After describing the neo-epitope process, it is time to zoom on the neo-epitope tTg/mTg antibodies in CD.

NEO-EPITOPE TISSUE TRANSGLUTAMINASE ANTIBODY IN THE DIAGNOSIS OF CELIAC DISEASE

In the last 2 decades reactivity to the neo-epitope tTg was explored in multiple studies, on various continents and in multiple countries, societies, and ethnicities, and gluten-dependent and gluten-independent diseases.[22,31,58,77–95] Many of the studies focused only on the neo-epitope tTg, but some compared its performance with other CD-associated serologic markers.[22,31,58,81,83] Summarizing those comparisons, it can be concluded that the neo-epitope tTg is a reliable diagnostic marker, at least

Table 3
Neo-epitope tTg check compared with IgA-tTg autoantibodies

No	Neo-Epitope tTg Check Advantages	IgA-tTg	References
1.	Covers IgA-deficient patients with CD	False-negative in IgA deficiency	22,58
2.	Average Sensitivity: >95%	>90%	22,31,58,81,83
3.	Average Specificity: >95%	>90%	22,31,58,81,83
4.	Intestinal damage reflection: +++	++	22,58
5.	Prediction of CD+++	++	78,79

comparable with the IgA-tTg, and may even outperform it.[22,31,58,81,83] Due to the high incidence of IgA deficiency in CD, most authors recommend measuring total IgA or to use the IgG isotype of the various antibodies if IgA deficiency were present. An additional advantage of the neo-epitope tTg is that its "check" version that includes the 2 isotypes, IgA + IgG.[22,58] **Table 3** summarizes the advantages of the neo-epitope tTg check over its IgA-tTg counterpart.

NEO-EPITOPE MICROBIAL TRANSGLUTAMINASE ANTIBODY IN THE DIAGNOSIS OF CELIAC DISEASE

Patients with CD can obtain mTg from their resident microbiome, as a processed food additive, from ingested probiotics, or infected nutrients or food.[68–71,96] As mentioned, it can deamidate or crosslink gliadin peptides resulting in an immunogenic complex, exposing a neo-epitope during the enzymatic reaction. It should be stressed that mTg is not an autoantibody because both its components are exogenous. However, its immunogenicity was reported in several studies[24,58] and recently presented at several international meetings. Specificities are 98%, 93%, and 87% for IgA, IgG, and check isotypes, respectively, and sensitivities are 64% to 65%, 94% to 95%, and 89% to 90% for IgA, IgG, and check isotypes, respectively.[24,58] The anti-neo-epitope mTg antibody isotypes are able to reflect CD intestinal pathology, and the IgG isotype reflects mucosal injury better than the IgA isotype. It seems that the neo-epitope mTg in CD is very specific, but with lower sensitivity; it is a new marker for the disease, reflects gut injury, but neo-epitope tTg outperforms the neo-epitope mTg antibodies in the diagnosis of CD.[97–99]

SUMMARY

Most patients affected by CD are asymptomatic or hyposymptomatic and undiagnosed and are at high risk of preventable complications, hence early correct diagnosis and gluten withdrawal are highly recommended. Multiple diagnostic antibodies are on the market. However, the older AGA and anti-DGP antibodies are losing popularity; the most frequently used are IgA-tTG and AEA. IgA-tTg has multiple false results and does not cover IgA deficiency. Anti-endomysium antibodies are less sensitive and interpretation is somewhat subjective. In the last 2 decades, a new generation of anti-neo-epitope tTg check (IgG + IgA) shows promise. It is highly sensitive and specific, covers IgA-deficient patients with CD, reflects intestinal damage, and has predictive potential in CD diagnosis.

REFERENCES

1. Moore LR. "But we're not hypochondriacs": the changing shape of gluten-free dieting and the contested illness experience. Soc Sci Med 2014;105:76–83.

2. Kim HS, Patel KG, Orosz E, et al. Time trends in the prevalence of celiac disease and gluten-free diet in the US population: results from the National Health and Nutrition Examination Surveys 2009-2014. JAMA Intern Med 2016;176:1716–7.

3. Turner JM. Diagnosis of celiac disease: taking a bite out of the controversy. Dig Dis Sci 2018;63:1384–91.

4. Lerner A, Jeremias P, Matthias T. The world incidence of celiac disease is increasing: a review. Int J Recent Sci Res 2015;7:5491–6.

5. Lerner A, Jeremias P, Matthias T. The world incidence and prevalence of autoimmune diseases is increasing: a review. Int J Celiac Disease 2015;3:151–5.

6. Lerner A. New therapeutic strategies for celiac disease. Autoimmun Rev 2010;9:144–7.

7. Lerner A, Agmon-Levin N, Shapira Y, et al. The thrombophilic network of autoantibodies in celiac disease. BMC Med 2013;11:89.

8. Lerner A, Matthias T. Extraintestinal manifestations of CD: common pathways in the gut-remote organs' axes. IntJ Celiac Dis 2017;5:24–7.

9. Lerner A, Matthias T. A silent or hypo-symptomatic disease can erupt: acute presentations of celiac disease. Int J Celiac Dis 2017;5:129–32.

10. Eliyah Livshits O, Shauol R, Reifen R, et al. Can celiac disease present along with childhood obesity? Int J Celiac Dis 2017;5:19–23.

11. Akman S, Şahaloğlu Ö, Dalkan C, et al. Is celiac disease misdiagnosed in children with functional constipation? Turk J Gastroenterol 2018;29:210–4.

12. Kelly D, Mearin ML, Ribes-Koninckx C. Paediatric coeliac disease: earlier diagnosis for better lifelong health. J Pediatr Gastroenterol Nutr 2018. https://doi.org/10.1097/MPG.0000000000002105.

13. Savilahti E, Viander M, Perkkiö M, et al. IgA antigliadin antibodies: a marker of mucosal damage in childhood coeliac disease. Lancet 1983;1(8320):320–2.

14. Tucker NT, Barghuthy FS, Prihoda TJ, et al. Antigliadin antibodies detected by enzyme-linked immunosorbent assay as a marker of childhood celiac disease. J Pediatr 1988;113:286–9.

15. Chorzelski TP, Sulej J, Tchorzewska H, et al. IgA class endomysium antibodies in dermatitis herpetiformis and coeliac disease. Ann N Y Acad Sci 1983;420:325–34.

16. Rossi TM, Kumar V, Lerner A, et al. Relationship of endomysial antibodies to jejunal mucosal pathology: specificity towards both symptomatic and asymptomatic celiacs. J Pediatr Gastroenterol Nutr 1988;7:858–63.

17. Dieterich W, Ehnis T, Bauer M, et al. Identification of tissue transglutaminase as the autoantigen of celiac disease. Nat Med 1997;3:797–801.

18. Dieterich W, Riecken EO, Schuppan D. Immunoassay for detection of IgA antitissue transglutaminase in patients with celiac disease. Methods Mol Med 2000;41:241–5.

19. Quarsten H, Molberg O, Fugger L, et al. HLA binding and T cell recognition of a tissue transglutaminase-modified gliadin epitope. Eur J Immunol 1999;29:2506–14.

20. Aleanzi M, Demonte AM, Esper C, et al. Celiac disease: antibody recognition against native and selectively deamidated gliadin peptides. Clin Chem 2001;47:2023–8.

21. Matthias T, Pfeiffer S, Selmi C, et al. Diagnostic challenges in celiac disease and the role of the tissue transglutaminase-neo-epitope. Clin Rev Allergy Immunol 2010;38:298–301.

22. Lerner A, Jeremias P, Neidhöfer S, et al. Antibodies against neo-epitope tTg complexed to gliadin are different and more reliable then anti-tTg for the diagnosis of pediatric celiac disease. J Immunol Methods 2016;429:15–20.
23. Lerner A, Matthias T. Microbial transglutaminase is a potential environmental inducer of celiac disease. In: Conrad K, Chan EKL, Andrade LEC, editors. From autoantibody research to standardized diagnostic assays in the management of human diseases. vol. 10, 12th symposium on autoantibodies. Dresden, Germany, September 23–26, 2015. p. 227–33. Pabst Science Publishers, Lengerich, Germany, e-pub.
24. Matthias T, Jeremias P, Neidhöfer S, et al. The industrial food additive microbial transglutaminase, mimics the tissue transglutaminase and is immunogenic in celiac disease patients. Autoimmun Rev 2016;15:1111–9.
25. Lerner A, Neidhöfer S, Matthias T. Serological markers and/or intestinal biopsies in the case-finding of celiac disease. Editorial. Int J Celiac Dis 2015;3:53–5.
26. Esteve M, Rosinach M, Llordés M, et al. Case-finding in primary care for coeliac disease: accuracy and cost-effectiveness of a rapid point-of-care test. United European Gastroenterol J 2018;6:855–65.
27. Elli L, Branchi F, Sidhu R, et al. Small bowel villous atrophy: celiac disease and beyond. Expert Rev Gastroenterol Hepatol 2017;11:125–38.
28. Lerner A, Matthias T. Intraepithelial lymphocyte normal cut-off level in celiac disease: the debate continues. Int J Celiac Dis 2016;4:4–6.
29. Marsh MN. It's counting that counts. Int J Celiac Dis 2016;4:1–3.
30. Peña AS. Counting intraepithelial lymphocytes. immunohistochemistry and flow cytometer are necessary new steps in the diagnosis of celiac disease. Int J Celiac Dis 2016;4:7–8.
31. Lerner A. Serological diagnosis of celiac disease – moving beyond the tip of the iceberg. Int J Celiac Dis 2014;2:64–6.
32. Husby S, Koletzko S, Korponay-Szabó IR, et al. European Society for Pediatric Gastroenterology, Hepatology, and Nutrition guidelines for the diagnosis of coeliac disease. J Pediatr Gastroenterol Nutr 2012;54:136–60.
33. Bishop J, Reed P, Austin P, et al. Prospective evaluation of the ESPGHAN guidelines for diagnosis of coeliac disease in New Zealand children. J Pediatr Gastroenterol Nutr 2018. https://doi.org/10.1097/MPG.0000000000002065.
34. Werkstetter KJ, Korponay-Szabó IR, Popp A, et al. Accuracy in diagnosis of celiac disease without biopsies in clinical practice. Gastroenterology 2017;153:924–35.
35. Holmes GKT, Forsyth JM, Knowles S, et al. Coeliac disease: further evidence that biopsy is not always necessary for diagnosis. Eur J Gastroenterol Hepatol 2017;29:640–5.
36. Wolf J, Petroff D, Richter T, et al. Validation of antibody-based strategies for diagnosis of pediatric celiac disease without biopsy. Gastroenterology 2017;153:410–9.e17.
37. Araya M, Díaz J, Oyarzun A, et al. Avoiding small intestinal biopsies for diagnosis of celiac disease in children: a reliable strategy for all patients? J Pediatr Gastroenterol Nutr 2018;66:785–8.
38. Lau MS, Sanders DS. Optimizing the diagnosis of celiac disease. Curr Opin Gastroenterol 2017;33:173–80.
39. Mills JR, Murray JA. Contemporary celiac disease diagnosis: is a biopsy avoidable? Curr Opin Gastroenterol 2016;32:80–5.
40. Freeman HJ. Role of biopsy in diagnosis and treatment of adult celiac disease. Gastroenterol Hepatol Bed Bench 2018;11:191–6.

41. Holmes G, Ciacci C. The serological diagnosis of coeliac disease - a step forward. Gastroenterol Hepatol Bed Bench 2018;11:209–15.
42. Marks LJ, Kurien M, Sanders DS. The serological diagnosis of adult coeliac disease - a cautious step forward? Gastroenterol Hepatol Bed Bench 2018;11: 175–7.
43. Smarrazzo A, Misak Z, Costa S, et al. Diagnosis of celiac disease and applicability of ESPGHAN guidelines in Mediterranean countries: a real life prospective study. BMC Gastroenterol 2017;17:17.
44. Samasca G, Sur G, Lupan L, et al. Challenges in the celiac disease diagnosis; Prague consensus. Gastroenterol Hepatol Bed Bench 2017;10:1–2.
45. Korponay-Szabó IR, Troncone R, Discepolo V. Adaptive diagnosis of coeliac disease. Best Pract Res Clin Gastroenterol 2015;29:381–98.
46. Kowalski K, Mulak A, Jasińska M, et al. Diagnostic challenges in celiac disease. Adv Clin Exp Med 2017;26:729–37.
47. Brusca I. Overview of biomarkers for diagnosis and monitoring of celiac disease. Adv Clin Chem 2015;68:1–55.
48. Leffler DA, Schuppan D. Update on serologic testing in celiac disease. Am J Gastroenterol 2010;105:2520–4.
49. Kumar V, Beutner EH, Lerner A, et al. Comparison of disease specificity of antiendomysial and antigliadin antibodies. In: Beutner EH, Chorzelski TP, Kumar V, editors. Immunopathology of the skin. New York: John Wiley; 1987. p. 483–8.
50. Kaswala DH, Veeraraghavan G, Kelly CP, et al. Celiac disease: diagnostic standards and dilemmas. Diseases 2015;3:86–101.
51. Lerner A, Kumar V, Iancu TC. Immunological diagnosis of childhood coeliac disease: comparison between antigliadin, antireticulin and antiendomysial antibodies. Clin Exp Immunol 1994;95:78–82.
52. Reif S, Lerner A. Tissue transglutaminase–the key player in celiac disease: a review. Autoimmun Rev 2004;3:40–5.
53. Lerner A, Neidhöfer S, Matthias T. Transglutaminase 2 and anti transglutaminase 2 autoantibodies in celiac disease and beyond: part A: TG2 double-edged sword: gut and extraintestinal involvement. Immunome Res 2015;11:101–5.
54. Lerner A, Neidhöfer S, Matthias T. Transglutaminase 2 and anti transglutaminase 2 autoantibodies in celiac disease and beyond. Part B: anti-transglutaminase 2 autoantibodies: friends or enemies. Immunome Res 2015;11:3–7.
55. Lerner A, Jeremias P, Matthias T. Outside of normal limits: false positive/negative anti TG2 autoantibodies. Int J Celiac Dis 2015;3:87–90.
56. Lerner A, Neidhöfer S, Matthias T. Anti-tTg-IgA is neither a solved problem nor a "closed case" in celiac disease diagnosis. Int J Celiac Dis 2017;5:97–100.
57. Hahn M, Hagel AF, Hirschmann S, et al. Modern diagnosis of celiac disease and relevant differential diagnoses in the case of cereal intolerance. Allergo J Int 2014;23:67–77.
58. Lerner A, Jeremias P, Neidhöfer S, et al. Comparison of the reliability of 17 celiac disease associated bio-markers to reflect intestinal damage. J Clin Cell Immunol 2017;8:1.
59. Lewis NR, Scott BB. Systematic review: the use of serology to exclude or diagnose coeliac disease (a comparison of the endomysial and tissue transglutaminase antibody tests). Aliment Pharmacol Ther 2006;24:47–54.
60. Hoerter NA, Shannahan SE, Suarez J, et al. Diagnostic yield of isolated deamidated gliadin peptide antibody elevation for celiac disease. Dig Dis Sci 2017; 62:1272–6.

61. Gould MJ, Brill H, Marcon MA, et al. In screening for celiac disease, deamidated gliadin rarely predicts disease when tissue transglutaminase is normal. J Pediatr Gastroenterol Nutr 2018. https://doi.org/10.1097/MPG.0000000000002109.

62. Zucchini L, Giusti D, Gatouillat G, et al. Interpretation of serological tests in the diagnosis of celiac disease: anti-deamidated gliadin peptide antibodies revisited. Autoimmunity 2016;49:414–20.

63. Sakly W, Mankaï A, Ghdess A, et al. Performance of anti-deamidated gliadin peptides antibodies in celiac disease diagnosis. Clin Res Hepatol Gastroenterol 2012;36:598–603.

64. Giersiepen K, Lelgemann M, Stuhldreher N, et al. Accuracy of diagnostic antibody tests for coeliac disease in children: summary of an evidence report. J Pediatr Gastroenterol Nutr 2012;54:229–41.

65. Mubarak A, Gmelig-Meyling FH, Wolters VM, et al. Immunoglobulin G antibodies against deamidated-gliadin-peptides outperform anti-endomysium and tissue transglutaminase antibodies in children <2 years age. APMIS 2011;119:894–900.

66. Brusca I, Carroccio A, Tonutti E, et al. The old and new tests for celiac disease: which is the best test combination to diagnose celiac disease in pediatric patients? Clin Chem Lab Med 2011;50:111–7.

67. Lewis NR, Scott BB. Meta-analysis: deamidated gliadin peptide antibody and tissue transglutaminase antibody compared as screening tests for coeliac disease. Aliment Pharmacol Ther 2010;31:73–81.

68. Lerner A, Aminov R, Matthias T. Dysbiosis may trigger autoimmune diseases via inappropriate posttranslational modification of host proteins. Front Microbiol 2016;7:84. Article 84.

69. Lerner A, Aminov R, Matthias T. Intestinal dysbiotic transglutaminases are potential environmental drivers of systemic autoimmunogenesis. Front Microbiol 2017; 8. article 66.

70. Lerner A, Matthias T. Possible association between celiac disease and bacterial transglutaminase in food processing: a hypothesis. Nutr Rev 2015;73:544–52.

71. Lerner A, Matthias T. Changes in intestinal tight junction permeability associated with industrial food additives explain the rising incidence of autoimmune disease. Autoimmun Rev 2015;14:479–89.

72. Matthias T, Neidhöfer S, Pfeiffer S, et al. Novel trends in celiac disease. Cell Mol Immunol 2011;8:121–5.

73. Mowat AM. Coeliac disease–a meeting point for genetics, immunology, and protein chemistry. Lancet 2003;361:1290–2.

74. Dieterich W, Esslinger B, Schuppan D. Pathomechanisms in celiac disease. Int Arch Allergy Immunol 2003;132:98–108.

75. Dewar D, Pereira SP, Ciclitira PJ. The pathogenesis of coeliac disease. Int J Biochem Cell Biol 2004;36:17–24.

76. Mackay IR, Rowley MJ. Autoimmune epitopes: autoepitopes. Autoimmun Rev 2004;3:487–92.

77. Barak M, Rozenberg O, Froom P, et al. Challenging our serological algorithm for celiac disease (CD) diagnosis by the ESPGHAN guidelines. Clin Chem Lab Med 2013;51:e257–9.

78. Bizzaro N, Tozzoli R, Villalta D, et al. Cutting-edge issues in celiac disease and in gluten intolerance. Clin Rev Allergy Immunol 2012;42:279–87.

79. Tozzoli R, Kodermaz G, Tampoia M, et al. Detection of autoantibodies specific for transglutaminase-gliadin peptides complex: a new way to explore the celiac iceberg. Riv Ital J Lab Med 2010;6:28–35.

80. Remes-Troche JM, Ramírez-Iglesias MT, Rubio-Tapia A, et al. Celiac disease could be a frequent disease in Mexico: prevalence of tissue transglutaminase antibody in healthy blood donors. J Clin Gastroenterol 2006;40:697–700.
81. Rozenberg O, Lerner A, Pacht A, et al. A new algorithm for the diagnosis of celiac disease. Cell Mol Immunol 2011;8:146–9.
82. Remes-Troche JM, Rios-Vaca A, Ramírez-Iglesias MT, et al. High prevalence of celiac disease in Mexican Mestizo adults with type 1 diabetes mellitus. J Clin Gastroenterol 2008;42:460–5.
83. Rozenberg O, Lerner A, Pacht A, et al. A novel algorithm for the diagnosis of celiac disease and a comprehensive review of celiac disease diagnostics. Clin Rev Allergy Immunol 2012;42:331–41.
84. Porcelli B, Ferretti F, Vindigni C, et al. Assessment of a test for the screening and diagnosis of celiac disease. J Clin Lab Anal 2014. https://doi.org/10.1002/jcla.21816.
85. Lytton SD, Antiga E, Pfeiffer S, et al. Neo-epitope tissue transglutaminase autoantibodies as a biomarker of the gluten sensitive skin disease–dermatitis herpetiformis. Clin Chim Acta 2013;415:346–9.
86. Lerner A, Neidhöfer S, Jeremias P, et al. The diversities between the neo-epitope and the IgA- tissue transglutaminase autoantibodies in celiac disease. In: Conrad K, Chan EKL, Andrade LEC, et al, editors. Autoantigens, autoantibodies, autoimmunity. Berlin, Germany: PABST Science Publishers; 2015. p. 220–6.
87. Ramakrishna BS, Makharia GK, Chetri K, et al. Prevalence of adult celiac disease in India: regional variations and associations. Am J Gastroenterol 2016;111:115–23.
88. Jenan M, Al Saffar J. Autoantibodies status in a sample of Iraqi celiac disease patients. Iraqi Journal of Science 2014;55:1259–63.
89. Rostami-Nejad M, Rostami K, Sanaei M, et al. Rotavirus and coeliac autoimmunity among adults with non-specific gastrointestinal symptoms. Saudi Med J 2010;31:891–4.
90. Hogen Esch CE, Wolters VM, Gerritsen SA, et al. Specific celiac disease antibodies in children on a gluten-free diet. Pediatrics 2011;128:547–52.
91. Mehrdad M, Mansour-Ghanaei F, Mohammadi F, et al. Frequency of celiac disease in patients with hypothyroidism. J Thyroid Res 2012;2012:201538.
92. Ganesh R, Suresh N, Sathiyasekaran Kanchi Kamakoti M. Celiac disease, still an uncommon problem in Tamilians? Indian J Gastroenterol 2009;28:189–91.
93. Dipper CR, Maitra S, Thomas R, et al. Anti-tissue transglutaminase antibodies in the follow-up of adult coeliac disease. Aliment Pharmacol Ther 2009;30:236–44.
94. Rostami Nejad M, Rostami K, Pourhoseingholi MA, et al. Atypical presentation is dominant and typical for coeliac disease. J Gastrointestin Liver Dis 2009;18:285–91.
95. Yap TW, Chan WK, Leow AH, et al. Prevalence of serum celiac antibodies in a multiracial Asian population - a first study in the young Asian adult population of Malaysia. PLoS One 2015;10:e0121908.
96. Lerner A, Aminov R, Matthias T. Horizontal gene transfer in the human gut. Front Immunol 2017;8. article 1630.
97. Matthias T, Lerner A. Microbial transglutaminase is immunogenic and potentially pathogenic in pediatric celiac disease. Front Pediatr 2018;6:389.
98. Lerner A, Matthias T. Microbial transglutaminase: a new potential player in celiac disease. Clin Immunol 2018. https://doi.org/10.1016/j.clim.2018.12.008.
99. Lerner A, Matthias T. Microbial transglutaminase is beneficial to food industries but a caveat to public health. Med One 2019;4:e190001.

Next Generation of Adeno-Associated Virus Vectors for Gene Therapy for Human Liver Diseases

Kenneth I. Berns, MD, PhD[a], Arun Srivastava, PhD[b,c],*

KEYWORDS

- AAV vectors • Gene transfer • Human liver diseases • Gene therapy

KEY POINTS

- The first generation of recombinant AAV vectors has shown efficacy in several phase I/II/III clinical trials targeting various human diseases, but the host immune response at high vector doses remains a challenge.
- The tissue-tropism of AAV vectors observed in animal models does not always correlate well with that in humans.
- A specific AAV serotype, AAV3, has been identified with which targeted delivery as well as high-efficiency transduction of human hepatocytes can be achieved.
- The next generation of AAV3 vectors has also been developed that is likely to circumvent most, if not all, of the problems associated with the first generation of AAV vectors in general.
- Further optimized AAV3 vectors should prove safe and effective for potential gene therapy for human liver diseases in general and hemophilia in particular.

Disclosure Statement: Dr K.I. Berns is a board member of Lacerta Therapeutics, a recently launched AAV gene therapy company. Dr A. Srivastava is a cofounder of, and holds equity in, Lacerta Therapeutics, aaVective, KASHX Bio, and Nirvana Therapeutics, and is an inventor on several issued patents on recombinant AAV vectors that have been licensed to various gene therapy companies.

[a] Department of Molecular Genetics and Microbiology, Powell Gene Therapy Center, University of Florida College of Medicine, Academic Research Building, Room R2-254, 1200 Newell Drive, Gainesville, FL 32610, USA; [b] Division of Cellular and Molecular Therapy, Department of Pediatrics, Powell Gene Therapy Center, Cancer and Genetics Research Complex, University of Florida College of Medicine, 2033 Mowry Road, Room 492-A, Gainesville, FL 32611, USA; [c] Division of Cellular and Molecular Therapy, Department of Molecular Genetics and Microbiology, Powell Gene Therapy Center, Cancer and Genetics Research Complex, University of Florida College of Medicine, 2033 Mowry Road, Room 492-A, Gainesville, FL 32611, USA
* Corresponding author. Division of Cellular and Molecular Therapy, Department of Pediatrics, Powell Gene Therapy Center, Cancer and Genetics Research Complex, University of Florida College of Medicine, 2033 Mowry Road, Room 492-A, Gainesville, FL 32611.
E-mail address: aruns@peds.ufl.edu

Gastroenterol Clin N Am 48 (2019) 319–330
https://doi.org/10.1016/j.gtc.2019.02.005
0889-8553/19/© 2019 Elsevier Inc. All rights reserved.

INTRODUCTION

Adeno-associated virus (AAV) is a small single-stranded (ss) DNA-containing nonpathogenic human parvovirus, which has gained attention as an efficient and safe vector for gene transfer.[1–6] Recombinant (r) AAV vectors have been, or currently are, used in 165 phase I/II/III clinical trials, and thus far, no serious adverse events have ever been observed or reported. AAV serotype 2 (AAV2) vectors have shown clinical efficacy in 3 human diseases: Leber congenital amaurosis,[7–10] aromatic L-amino acid decarboxylase deficiency,[11] and choroideremia.[12] In the past decade, at least 12 additional AAV serotype vectors, some derived from nonhuman primates (NHPs), have also become available.[13–21] AAV1 vectors have successfully been used in the gene therapy for lipoprotein lipase deficiency,[22] and AAV serotype 8 (AAV8) vectors have shown clinical efficacy in the potential gene therapy for hemophilia B.[23–25] More recently, AAV serotype 2 (AAV5) vectors have been effective in hemophilia A.[26,27] AAV serotype 9 (AAV9) vectors have successfully been used in gene therapy for Pompe disease[28] and in spinal muscular atrophy.[29] The AAV serotype 1 (AAV1)-Lipoprotein lipase (LPL) vector was approved as a drug, designated as alipogene tiparvovec, and marketed under the trade name (Glybera, uniQure, Amsterdam), in Europe in 2012, although it was withdrawn in 2017. In 2017, an AAV2 vector expressing retinal pigment epithelium–specific 65 kDa protein was approved by the Food and Drug Administration as a drug, voretigene neparvovec (Luxturna, Spark Therapeutics, Philadelphia), in the United States. Several additional phase I/II clinical trials have been, or currently are, pursued with AAV1, AAV2, AAV serotype 3 (AAV3), AAV5, AAV serotype 6, AAV8, AAV9, and AAV serotype 10 vectors for potential gene therapy for a wide variety of human diseases.[30]

Despite these remarkable achievements, it has become increasingly clear that the full potential of the first generation of AAV vectors will be realized only after these vectors have been modified to evade the host immune response.[31] A brief account of the use of AAV vectors in targeting the liver in general, and gene therapy for hemophilia in particular, follows.

LIVER-TROPIC ADENO-ASSOCIATED VIRUS VECTORS

Liver has long been considered among the ideal targets for potential gene therapy for a wide variety of human diseases. In 1997, Ponnazhagan and colleagues[32] first reported the liver-tropism of rAAV2 vectors, after intravenous administration of rAAV2-lacZ vectors, in a murine model in vivo. Koeberl and colleagues[33] and Snyder and colleagues[34] documented persistent expression of human clotting factor IX (F.IX) after intravenous injection in mice as well. Subsequently, persistent expression of canine factor IX in hemophilia B canines was also reported by Chao and colleagues.[35] Based on those preclinical studies, a phase I clinical trial for hemophilia B was carried out with AAV2 vectors expressing hF.IX.[35] Even though in preclinical studies with both hemophilic murine and canine models, rAAV2-F.IX vectors provided complete phenotypic correction of the disease for the entire life spans of these animals, the predicted dose of these vectors in humans did not express therapeutic levels of F.IX in humans. The results of the first phase I clinical trial for potential gene therapy for hemophilia B with the first generation of rAAV2 vectors were reported in 2006.[36] At low (8×10^{10} vector genomes [vgs]/kg) and medium (4×10^{11} vgs/kg) vector doses, rAAV2 vectors failed to express F.IX in 2 patients. At the high dose (2×10^{12} vgs/kg), rAAV2 vectors did lead to expression of therapeutic levels of F.IX in 1 patient, but it was short-lived due to the host immune response to AAV2 capsid proteins. Uptake of AAV2 vectors by dendritic cells, followed by proteasomal degradation of capsid proteins, led to activation of AAV2 capsid-specific CD8$^+$ memory T cells, which in turn, led to the destruction of transduced hepatocytes and, consequently, the loss of F.IX levels in this patient.[37] The lesson learned from this first liver-directed gene therapy trial was that AAV2 serotype vectors, although extremely effective in mice and dogs, were not optimal for humans.

In the ensuing years, several additional AAV serotype vectors became available, and their tissue/organ tropisms were determined.[13–21,38] The 10 most commonly used AAV serotype vectors are depicted schematically in **Fig. 1**A. Several investigators reported remarkably high efficiency of transduction of murine liver with AAV8 serotype vectors.[18,39,40] A subsequent clinical trial with AAV8 vectors, performed by Nathwani and colleagues,[23] proved a significant step forward, but a similar immune response also was observed in the high-dose cohort of patients.[24] Although the choice of AAV8 vector undoubtedly was based on its superior performance over AAV2 vectors in transducing murine hepatocytes, it was not readily apparent whether AAV8 vectors would be ideal for transducing human hepatocytes. This question proved particularly difficult to address because AAV8 failed to transduce any cell type, including hepatocytes in vitro.

SELECTIVE HUMAN LIVER TROPISM OF ADENO-ASSOCIATED VIRUS SEROTYPE 3 VECTORS

In the quest to identify an alternative AAV serotype for efficient transduction of human hepatocytes, Glushakova and colleagues[41] made an unexpected observation approximately a decade ago that AAV3 vectors, shown schematically in **Fig. 1**B, could

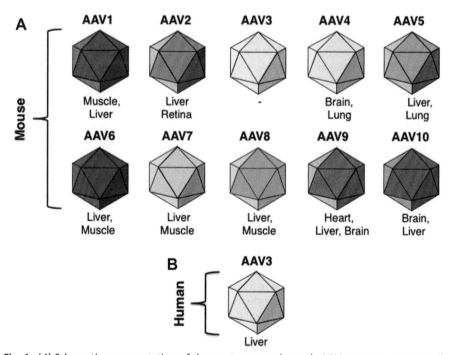

Fig. 1. (*A*) Schematic representation of the most commonly used rAAV serotype vectors and their tissue-tropism. Various murine tissues and organs that have been reported to be transduced efficiently with various AAV serotype vectors are indicated. (*B*) AAV3 serotype vectors in particular, have been shown to transduce human hepatocytes well. (*Data from* Refs.[41–44,47,48,62])

efficiently transduce human liver cancer cell lines as well as primary human hepatocytes efficiently in vitro. Cheng and colleagues[42] and Ling and colleagues[43] documented that human liver tumors also could be transduced remarkably well in xenograft mouse model in vivo. Ling and colleagues[44] provided the underlying basis of the remarkable tropism of AAV3 vectors for human hepatic cells because AAV3 uses human hepatocyte growth factor receptor (huHGFR) as a cellular coreceptor. Although murine hepatocyte growth factor receptor (muHGFR) shares 88% identity with huHGFR,[44] 44 AAV3 fails to bind to muHGFR because of the location of amino acid differences along the interaction interface, including amino residues that make contact with hepatocyte growth factor. Lisowski and colleagues[45] reported that a shuffled rAAV vector, designated LK-03, which shares 97.7% and 98.9% homology with rAAV3B at the DNA and amino acids level, respectively, transduced human primary hepatocytes approximately 20-fold more efficiently than AAV8.

ADENO-ASSOCIATED VIRUS SEROTYPE 3 AND NONHUMAN PRIMATE STUDIES

Although murine xenograft mouse models, used by Cheng and colleagues[42] and Ling and colleagues,[43] provided a useful system to evaluate the efficacy of AAV3 vectors in human hepatocyte transduction, the safety of these vectors could not be assessed in such models because AAV3 vectors do not transduce any tissues or organs in mice,[46] and because of the close phylogenetic and physiologic similarities between NHPs and humans. The safety and efficacy of rAAV3 vectors were evaluated by Li and colleagues[47] in an NHP model in vivo. The human and the NHP hepatocyte growth factor receptors (HGFRs) share 99% identity. High-efficiency transduction of NHP livers, both short term (7 days) and long term (91 days), after intravenous delivery of rAAV3 vectors, was documented, with no apparent toxicity at a relatively high dose of 1×10^{13} vgs/kg. These findings revealed the efficient liver-targeted gene transfer by rAAV3 vectors after systematic administration. Remarkably, the vector-mediated enhanced green fluorescent protein (EGFP) expression and vector genome accumulation were largely restricted to the NHP liver. Although the use of the EGFP reporter gene allowed the authors to address both vector tropism and gene transfer efficiency simultaneously, it was less quantitative and likely immunogenic, leading to transient expression. The use of a secreted self-antigen, rhesus chorionic gonadotropin (rhCG), allowed the authors to study not only the efficiency but also the onset and kinetics of transgene expression and long-term stability. In addition, because the rhCG used in this study can limit the potential host humoral and cellular immune responses to the transgene product, the authors were also able to evaluate the potential host immune responses against the vector capsid proteins for up to 3 months. The vector genome biodistribution study clearly revealed that the persisting vector genomes of rAAV3 vectors were predominantly harbored in the monkey liver. Furthermore, the rhCG mRNA expression pattern in 6 selected organs displayed that the transgene expression was largely restricted to the liver, which also did not lead to any overt cytotoxicity. In addition, no obvious vector-related pathologic changes in the liver, spleen, and other organs were observed in any of the treated animals. These studies documented the remarkable specificity, efficacy, and safety of rAAV3 vectors in NHP livers after systemic administration. These studies were further corroborated by Wang and colleagues,[48] which further established the remarkable specificity, efficacy, and safety of AAV3 vectors.[4]

NEXT GENERATION OF ADENO-ASSOCIATED VIRUS VECTORS

Hansen and colleagues[49] made the original observation that after infection of cells, only approximately 20% of the input AAV2 vectors gain entry into the nucleus, whereas approximately 80% fail to escape the endosome in the cytoplasm. It was subsequently reported by Duan and colleagues[50] that AAV2 capsids become ubiquitinated in the cytoplasm, where they are targeted for degradation by the host cell proteasomal machinery, thereby having a negative impact on the transduction efficiency of the first generation of AAV vectors. One of the major obstacles that limit the transduction efficiency of AAV vectors in general is ubiquitination, followed by proteasomal-mediated degradation. Previously, Mah and colleagues[51] had observed that inhibition of the host cell EGFR protein tyrosine kinase (EGFR-PTK) resulted in a significant increase in the transduction efficiency of AAV2 vectors. Thus, it was hypothesized that after infection, the AAV2 capsid protein becomes phosphorylated at surface-exposed tyrosine residues by EGFR-PTK and that tyrosine phosphorylation leads to ubiquitination, followed by proteasomal degradation of AAV2 vectors in the cytoplasm.[50,52] Zhong and colleagues[53] provided experimental evidence in 2007 to support this hypothesis. These studies provided the impetus to mutagenize the surface-exposed tyrosine residues in the AAV2 capsid to circumvent this barrier.

There are 7 tyrosine (Y) residues in the AAV2 capsid that are surface-exposed (Y252, Y272, Y444, Y500, Y700, Y704, and Y730). Each of these Y residues was mutagenized by Zhong and colleagues[54] to phenylalanine (F) residues to generate 7 single mutants (Y252F, Y272F, Y444F, Y500F, Y700F, Y704F, and Y730F), the transduction efficiency of 3 of which (Y444F, Y500F, and Y730F) was significantly higher than their wild-type (WT) counterpart.[55] The Y730F single-mutant AAV2 vector was the most efficient, the use of which resulted in the expression of therapeutic levels of hF.IX in 3 different strains of mice after intravenous or portal vein administration at 10-fold reduced vector doses.[54] When the 3 most efficient mutations were combined into 1 capsid, the resulting triple-mutant (Y444+500+730F) vectors showed a further 3-fold increase in F.IX expression in hemophilia B mice.[55] Furthermore, this triple-mutant AAV2 vector was shown to minimizes in vivo targeting of transduced hepatocytes by capsid-specific CD8[+] T cells.[56]

In the quest to develop more efficient and potentially less immunogenic AAV vectors, these studies were extended to include 2 additional amino acid residues in the AAV capsid that are surface exposed and also can be phosphorylated by cellular serine/threonine protein kinases. For example, in addition to 7 tyrosine (Y) residues, the AAV2 capsid contains 17 surface-exposed serine (S) and 15 surface-exposed threonine (T) residues, each of which was mutagenized, and AAV2 vectors containing various permutations and combinations thereof, depicted schematically in **Fig. 2A**, were generated.[57,58] In addition, because ubiquitination occurs on lysine (K) residues, all 7 surface-exposed residues in the AAV2 capsid were mutagenized, and a limited number of Y+S+T+K–mutant AAV2 vectors were generated.[59]

Most, if not all, of the surface-exposed Y, S, T, and K residues, however, are highly conserved among all 10 commonly used AAV serotype vectors, and most of these residues also have been mutagenized in each of 10 AAV serotype vectors. The corresponding Y–, S–, T–, and K– mutants of AAV3 vectors also are shown in **Fig. 2A**. A quadruple-mutant (Y444+500+730F+T491V) for AAV2, and a double-mutant (S663V+T492V) for AAV3, shown schematically in **Fig. 2B**, have been identified to be the most efficient in transducing the normal and murine xenograft models, respectively.[60]

In addition to the WT AAV3 vectors, Li and colleagues[47] evaluated the safety and efficacy of the S663V+T492V double-mutant AAV3 (AAV3-ST) vectors in NHPs. The results revealed that the transduction efficiency of this capsid-modified vector was approximately 5-fold higher compared with its WT counterpart, with no apparent vector-related toxicity. Thus, the use of capsid-modified next generation of AAV

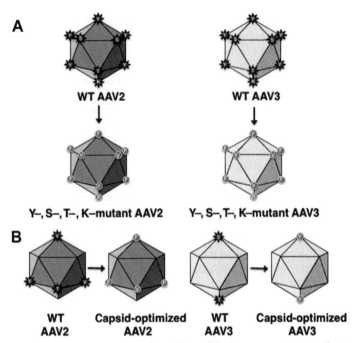

Fig. 2. (*A*) Schematic representation of capsid-modified next generation of rAAV vectors. Surface-exposed, specific tyrosine (Y), serine (S), and threonine (T) residues on AAV capsids can be phosphorylated, which is a signal for ubiquitination. Surface-exposed, specific lysine (K) residues on AAV capsids can be ubiquitinated and subsequently degraded by the host cell proteasome machinery. Site-directed mutagenesis of these residues leads to the generation of AAV vectors that are more efficient at reduced vector doses and, consequently, less immunogenic. (*B*) Specific examples of the most efficient AAV2,[54–56,58,60] and AAV3,[42,43,47,60,62] serotype vectors generated thus far are also depicted.

vectors is likely to overcome some of the limitations associated with the first generation of AAV vectors.

ADENO-ASSOCIATED VIRUS 3 VECTORS AND HUMANIZED MOUSE MODELS

In 2014, Lisowski and colleagues[45] reported that a shuffled rAAV vector, designated LK-03, which shares 97.7% and 98.9% homology with rAAV3 at the DNA and amino acids level, respectively, transduced human primary hepatocytes in a humanized mouse model in vivo, and it was approximately 20-fold more efficient than AAV8. In studies performed by Li and colleagues[47] with a different humanized liver xenograft mouse model,[61] it was observed that AAV3 was approximately 12-fold more efficient than AAV8 in transducing human hepatocytes in vivo.[14] In a more recent study, Vercauteren and colleagues[62] compared the transduction efficiencies of AAV3-ST vectors with AAV8 and AAV5 vectors that are currently used in gene therapy for hemophilia (**Table 1**). In this humanized mouse model, it was reported that rAAV3-ST vectors were approximately 8 times more efficient than rAAV8 vectors, and approximately 82 times more efficient than rAAV5 vectors in transducing primary human hepatocytes.[62] Although the ultimate efficacy of AAV3 vectors will only be revealed by clinical trials in humans, it seems likely that these vectors will prove safer and more efficient than AAV8 and AAV5 vectors in targeting human liver diseases in general and gene therapy for hemophilia in particular.

Table 1
First generation of recombinant adeno-associated virus serotype vectors used/being used for potential gene therapy for hemophilia

	Investigators/Sponsors	Vector	Dose	Expression Level	Total Dose[a]	Ref.
Hemophilia B	High/Kay	ssAAV2	8×10^{10} vgs/kg	0%	5.6 trillion	Manno et al,[36] 2006
			4×10^{11} vgs/kg	0%	28 trillion	
			2×10^{12} vgs/kg	11%→0%	140 trillion	
	Nathwani/Davidoff	scAAV8	2×10^{11} vgs/kg	2%	14 trillion	Nathwani et al,[24] 2014, and George et al,[25] 2017
			6×10^{11} vgs/kg	2%–4%	42 trillion	
			2×10^{12} vgs/kg	8%–12% → 5%	140 trillion	
	Baxalta[b]	scAAV8	2×10^{11} vgs/kg	2%–5%	14 trillion	Terry[64] and Herzog,[68] 2016
			1×10^{12} vgs/kg	20%–25%	70 trillion	
			3×10^{12} vgs/kg	50% → ?%	210 trillion	
	Spark Therapeutics	Modified ssAAV8	5×10^{11} vgs/kg	28%–41% → 26%–33%	35 trillion	George et al,[25] 2017
	Dimension Therapeutics[c]	ssAAVrh10	1.6×10^{12} vgs/kg	<2%	112 trillion	Semedo[65]
			3×10^{12} vgs/kg	<2%	210 trillion	
	uniQure	scAAV5	5×10^{12} vgs/kg	3%–6.8%	350 trillion	Miesbach et al,[26] 2018
			2×10^{13} vgs/kg	3%–12.7%	1.4 quadrillion	
Hemophilia A	BioMarin	ssAAV5	2×10^{13} vgs/kg	2%–5%	1.4 quadrillion	Rangarajan et al,[27] 2017, and Gatlin[66]
			6×10^{13} vgs/kg	50%–200% → 32%–59%	4.2 quadrillion	
	Spark Therapeutics	ssLK-03	5×10^{11} vgs/kg	6%–37%	35 trillion	Pagliarulo[67]
			1×10^{12} vgs/kg	7%–24%	70 trillion	
			2×10^{12} vgs/kg	16%–49%[d]	140 trillion	

[a] Based on an average patient's weight of 70 kg (estimated number of cells in a 70-kg reference man = 3×10^{13}, or 30 trillion).[69]
[b] Acquired by Shire.
[c] Acquired by Ultragenyx.
[d] Serious adverse events in 2 patients.

GENE THERAPY FOR HEMOPHILIA WITH ADENO-ASSOCIATED VIRUS VECTORS

Table 1 lists all clinical trials in which various AAV serotypes and their variants that have been used, or are currently, used in potential gene therapy for both hemophilia B and hemophilia A. As stated previously, after the short-lived expression hF.IX mediated by the first-generation AAV2 vectors,[37] the use of AAV8 vectors proved successful.[23] The hF.IX levels declined, however, from approximately 8% to 12% to approximately 5% over a 3-year follow-up period.[24] Although the superior performance of AAV8 vectors in humans seemed parallel that observed in murine models, the vector genome used was double-stranded self-complementary (sc), in contrast to that used in the first clinical trial with AAV2 vectors, which was single-stranded, and ssAAV DNA is known to transcriptionally inactive and viral second-strand DNA synthesis is known to be a rate-limiting step during AAV vector-mediated transgene expression.[63] Thus, it seems that the use of scAAV genome, rather than the AAV8 serotype, contributed to the successful outcome because AAV8 vectors transduce human hepatocytes less efficiently than mouse hepatocytes.[47,48,62] The next trial, sponsored by Baxalta, also with scAAV8 vectors, yielded inconsistent results, and, as a consequence, this trial was halted.[64] The trial sponsored by (Spark Therapeutics, Philadelphia, USA), however, using a capsid-modified ssAAV vector, has led to therapeutic levels of hF.IX at relatively low doses.[25] The trial sponsored by (Dimension Therapeutics, Boston, Massachusetts) using ssAAVrhesus10 vectors failed to lead to expression therapeutic levels of hF.IX, even at significantly high doses and, as a consequence, this trial was also halted.[65] Using scAAV5 vectors, uniQure recently reported modest levels of expression of hF.IX; however, enormously high vector doses were required[26] (see **Table 1**).

The results of 2 phase I clinical trials for gene therapy for hemophilia A also been have reported. In the BioMarin-sponsored trial with ssAAV5 vectors, human clotting Factor VIII (h.FVIII) levels ranging from approximately 50% to 200% were achieved.[27] There has been a steady decline, however, over time, ranging between approximately 32% and 59%.[66] More recently, Spark Therapeutics reported that with the use of ssLK-03, a shuffled ssAAV vector with significant homology to AAV3, h.FVIII levels ranging from approximately 16% to 49% were achieved, but at the highest vector dose, 2 patients experienced severe adverse events.[67]

Taken together, the following conclusions can be drawn: (1) the tropism, safety, and efficacy of AAV vectors in animal models do not necessarily translate well in humans; (2) the use of AAV vectors composed of naturally occurring capsids is likely to induce immune responses, especially at high doses because the host immune system cannot distinguish between AAV as a virus versus AAV as a vector; (3) the host immune response is directly correlated with the AAV vector dose; and (4) because the WT AAV did not evolve for the purposes of delivery of therapeutic genes, rAAV vectors composed of naturally occurring capsid are unlikely to be optimal in human clinical trials.[31] Overall, the authors' prediction is that, in contrast to the high vector doses that currently are used with AAV8 and AAV5 vectors for hemophilia B and hemophilia A, respectively, the optimized AAV3 serotype vectors, in addition to being far more efficacious, will offer potential advantages of being less immunogenic and more cost-effective for their use in human liver diseases in general and in hemophilia in particular.[4]

ACKNOWLEDGMENTS

The authors gratefully acknowledge their colleagues and collaborators, both past and present, for helpful scientific discussions. This work was supported in part by

Public Health Service grants R01 HL-097088, R41 AI-122735, and R21 EB-015684 from the National Institutes of Health; a grant from the Children's Miracle Network; and support from the Kitzman Foundation.

REFERENCES

1. Samulski RJ, Muzyczka N. AAV-mediated gene therapy for research and therapeutic purposes. Annu Rev Virol 2014;1:427–51.
2. Muzyczka N, Berns KI. AAV's golden jubilee. Mol Ther 2015;23:807–8.
3. Grimm D, Zolotukhin SE. Pluribus unum: 50 years of research, millions of viruses, and one goal - tailored acceleration of AAV evolution. Mol Ther 2015;23:1819–31.
4. Srivastava A. Advances and challenges in the use of recombinant adeno-associated virus vectors for human gene therapy. Cell Gene Ther Insights 2016;2:553–75.
5. Berns KI, Muzyczka N. AAV: an overview of unanswered questions. Hum Gene Ther 2017;28:308–13.
6. Weinmann J, Grimm D. Next-generation AAV vectors for clinical use: an ever-accelerating race. Virus Genes 2017;53:707–13.
7. Bainbridge JW, Smith AJ, Barker SS, et al. Effect of gene therapy on visual function in Leber's congenital amaurosis. N Engl J Med 2008;358:2231–9.
8. Maguire AM, Simonelli F, Pierce EA, et al. Safety and efficacy of gene transfer for Leber's congenital amaurosis. N Engl J Med 2008;358:2240–8.
9. Cideciyan AV, Aleman TS, Boye SL, et al. Human gene therapy for RPE65 isomerase deficiency activates the retinoid cycle of vision but with slow rod kinetics. Proc Natl Acad Sci U S A 2008;105:15112–7.
10. Hauswirth WW, Aleman TS, Kaushal S, et al. Treatment of Leber congenital amaurosis due to RPE65 mutations by ocular subretinal injection of adeno-associated virus gene vector: Short-term results of a phase I trial. Hum Gene Ther 2008;19: 979–90.
11. Hwu WL, Muramatsu S, Tseng SH, et al. Gene therapy for aromatic L-amino acid decarboxylase deficiency. Sci Transl Med 2012;4:134ra61.
12. MacLaren RE, Groppe M, Barnard AR, et al. Retinal gene therapy in patients with choroideremia: Initial findings from a phase 1/2 clinical trial. Lancet 2014;383: 1129–37.
13. Xiao W, Chirmule N, Berta SC, et al. Gene therapy vectors based on adeno-associated virus type 1. J Virol 1999;73:3994–4003.
14. Muramatsu S, Mizukami H, Young NS, et al. Nucleotide sequencing and generation of an infectious clone of adeno-associated virus 3. Virology 1996;221: 208–17.
15. Chiorini JA, Yang L, Liu Y, et al. Cloning of adeno-associated virus type 4 (AAV4) and generation of recombinant AAV4 particles. J Virol 1997;71:6823–33.
16. Bantel-Schaal U, Delius H, Schmidt R, et al. Human adeno-associated virus type 5 is only distantly related to other known primate helper-dependent parvoviruses. J Virol 1999;73:939–47.
17. Rutledge EA, Halbert CL, Russell DW. Infectious clones and vectors derived from adeno-associated virus (AAV) serotypes other than AAV type 2. J Virol 1998;72: 309–19.
18. Gao GP, Alvira MR, Wang L, et al. Novel adeno-associated viruses from rhesus monkeys as vectors for human gene therapy. Proc Natl Acad Sci U S A 2002; 99:11854–9.

19. Mori S, Wang L, Takeuchi T, et al. Two novel adeno-associated viruses from cynomolgus monkey: pseudotyping characterization of capsid protein. Virol 2004; 330:375–83.

20. Schmidt M, Voutetakis A, Afione S, et al. Adeno-associated virus type 12 (AAV12): A novel AAV serotype with sialic acid- and heparan sulfate proteoglycan-independent transduction activity. J Virol 2008;82:1399–406.

21. Schmidt M, Govindasamy L, Afione S, et al. Molecular characterization of the heparin-dependent transduction domain on the capsid of a novel adeno-associated virus isolate, AAV(VR-942). J Virol 2008;82:8911–6.

22. Gaudet D, Methot J, Dery S, et al. Efficacy and long-term safety of alipogene tiparvovec (AAV1-LPL^{s447x}) gene therapy for lipoprotein lipase deficiency: an open-label trial. Gene Ther 2013;20:361–9.

23. Nathwani AC, Tuddenham EG, Rangarajan S, et al. Adenovirus-associated virus vector-mediated gene transfer in hemophilia B. N Engl J Med 2011;365:2357–65.

24. Nathwani AC, Reiss UM, Tuddenham EG, et al. Long-term safety and efficacy of factor IX gene therapy in hemophilia B. N Engl J Med 2014;371:1994–2004.

25. George LA, Sullivan SK, Giermasz JEJ, et al. Hemophilia B gene therapy with a high-specific-activity factor IX variant. N Engl J Med 2017;377:2215–27.

26. Miesbach W, Meijer K, Coppens M, et al. Gene therapy with adeno-associated virus vector 5-human factor IX in adults with hemophilia B. Blood 2018;131: 1022–31.

27. Rangarajan S, Walsh L, Lester W, et al. AAV5-factor VIII gene transfer in severe hemophilia A. N Engl J Med 2017;377:2519–30.

28. Byrne PI, Collins S, Mah CS, et al. Phase I/II trial of diaphragm delivery of recombinant adeno-associated virus acid alpha-glucosidase (rAAV1-CMV-GAA) gene vector in patients with Pompe disease. Hum Gene Ther Clin Dev 2014;25:134–63.

29. Mendell JR, Al-Zaidy S, Shell R, et al. Single-dose gene-replacement therapy for spinal muscular atrophy. N Engl J Med 2017;377:1713–22.

30. Ling C, Zhong L, Srivastava A. Adeno-associated viral vectors in gene therapy. Chichester (United Kingdom): eLS John Wiley & Sons, Ltd; 2018.

31. Srivastava A. Adeno-associated virus: the naturally occurring virus versus the recombinant vector. Hum Gene Ther 2016;27(1):1–6.

32. Ponnazhagan S, Mukherjee P, Yoder MC, et al. Adeno-associated virus 2-mediated gene transfer in vivo: organ-tropism and expression of transduced sequences in mice. Gene 1997;190:203–10.

33. Koeberl DD, Alexander IE, Halbert CL, et al. Persistent expression of human clotting factor IX from mouse liver after intravenous injection of adeno-associated virus vectors. Proc Natl Acad Sci U S A 1997;94:1426–31.

34. Snyder RO, Miao CH, Patijn GA, et al. Persistent and therapeutic concentrations of human factor IX in mice after hepatic gene transfer of recombinant AAV vectors. Nat Genet 1997;16:270–6.

35. Chao H, Samulski R, Bellinger D, et al. Persistent expression of canine factor IX in hemophilia B canines. Gene Ther 1990;6:1695–704.

36. Manno CS, Pierce GF, Arruda VR, et al. Successful transduction of liver in hemophilia by AAV-factor IX and limitations imposed by the host immune response. Nat Med 2006;12:342–7.

37. Mingozzi F, Maus MV, Hui DJ, et al. CD8$^{(+)}$ T-cell responses to adeno-associated virus capsid in humans. Nat Med 2007;13:419–22.

38. Srivastava A. In vivo tissue-tropism of adeno-associated viral vectors. Curr Opin Virol 2016;21:75–80.

39. Sarkar R, Tetreault R, Gao G, et al. Total correction of hemophilia A mice with canine FVIII using an AAV8 serotype. Blood 2004;103:1253–60.
40. Thomas CE, Storm TA, Huang Z, et al. Rapid uncoating of vector genomes is the key to efficient liver transduction with pseudotyped adeno-associated virus vectors. J Virol 2004;78:3110–22.
41. Glushakova LG, Lisankie MJ, Eruslanov EB, et al. AAV3-mediated transfer and expression of the pyruvate dehydrogenase E1 alpha subunit gene causes metabolic remodeling and apoptosis of human liver cancer cells. Mol Genet Metab 2009;98:289–99.
42. Cheng B, Ling C, Dai Y, et al. Development of optimized AAV3 serotype vectors: Mechanism of high-efficiency transduction of human liver cancer cells. Gene Ther 2012;19:375–84.
43. Ling C, Wang Y, Zhang Y, et al. Selective in vivo targeting of human liver tumors by optimized AAV3 vectors in a murine xenograft model. Hum Gene Ther 2014; 25(12):1023–34.
44. Ling C, Lu Y, Kalsi JK, et al. Human hepatocyte growth factor receptor is a cellular coreceptor for adeno-associated virus serotype 3. Hum Gene Ther 2010;21(12): 1741–7.
45. Lisowski L, Dane AP, Chu K, et al. Selection and evaluation of clinically relevant AAV variants in a xenograft liver model. Nature 2014;506(7488):382–6.
46. Zincarelli C, Soltys S, Rengo G, et al. Analysis of AAV serotypes 1-9 mediated gene expression and tropism in mice after systemic injection. Mol Ther 2008; 16(6):1073–80.
47. Li S, Ling C, Zhong L, et al. Efficient and targeted transduction of nonhuman primate liver with systemically delivered optimized AAV3b vectors. Mol Ther 2015; 23(12):1867–76.
48. Wang L, Bell P, Somanathan S, et al. Comparative study of liver gene transfer with AAV vectors based on natural and engineered AAV capsids. Mol Ther 2015; 23(12):1877–87.
49. Hansen J, Qing K, Kwon HJ, et al. Impaired intracellular trafficking of adeno-associated virus type 2 vectors limits efficient transduction of murine fibroblasts. J Virol 2000;74(2):992–6.
50. Duan D, Yue Y, Yan Z, et al. Endosomal processing limits gene transfer to polarized airway epithelia by adeno-associated virus. J Clin Invest 2000;105(11): 1573–87.
51. Mah C, Qing K, Khuntirat B, et al. Adeno-associated virus type 2-mediated gene transfer: Role of epidermal growth factor receptor protein tyrosine kinase in transgene expression. J Virol 1998;72(12):9835–43.
52. Zhong L, Li B, Jayandharan G, et al. Tyrosine-phosphorylation of AAV2 vectors and its consequences on viral intracellular trafficking and transgene expression. Virology 2008;381(2):194–202.
53. Zhong L, Zhao W, Wu J, et al. A dual role of EGFR protein tyrosine kinase signaling in ubiquitination of AAV2 capsids and viral second-strand DNA synthesis. Mol Ther 2007;15:1323–30.
54. Zhong L, Li B, Mah CS, et al. Next generation of adeno-associated virus 2 vectors: Point mutations in tyrosines lead to high-efficiency transduction at lower doses. Proc Natl Acad Sci U S A 2008;105:7827–32.
55. Markusic DM, Herzog RW, Aslanidi GV, et al. High-efficiency transduction and correction of murine hemophilia B using AAV2 vectors devoid of multiple surface-exposed tyrosines. Mol Ther 2010;18:2048–56.

56. Martino AT, Basner-Tschakarjan E, Markusic DM, et al. Engineered AAV vector minimizes in vivo targeting of transduced hepatocytes by capsid-specific CD8+ T cells. Blood 2013;121:2224–33.

57. Aslanidi GV, Rivers AE, Ortiz L, et al. High-efficiency transduction of human monocyte-derived dendritic cells by capsid-modified recombinant AAV2 vectors. Vaccine 2012;30:3908–17.

58. Aslanidi GV, Rivers AE, Ortiz L, et al. Optimization of the capsid of recombinant adeno-associated virus 2 (AAV2) vectors: the final threshold? PLoS One 2013; 8:e59142.

59. Li B, Ma W, Ling C, et al. Site-directed mutagenesis of surface-exposed lysine residues leads to improved transduction by AAV2, but Not AAV8, vectors in murine hepatocytes in vivo. Hum Gene Ther Methods 2015;26:211–20.

60. Ling C, Li B, Ma W, et al. Development of optimized AAV serotype vectors for high-efficiency transduction at further reduced doses. Hum Gene Ther Methods 2016;27:143–9.

61. Borel F, Tang Q, Gernoux G, et al. Survival advantage of both human hepatocyte xenografts and genome-edited hepatocytes for treatment of α-1 antitrypsin deficiency. Mol Ther 2017;25:2477–89.

62. Vercauteren K, Hoffman BE, Zolotukhin I, et al. Superior in vivo transduction of human hepatocytes using engineered AAV3 capsid. Mol Ther 2016;24:1042–9.

63. McCarty DM, Monahan PE, Samulski RJ. Self-complementary recombinant adeno-associated virus (scAAV) vectors promote efficient transduction independently of DNA synthesis. Gene Ther 2001;8:1248–54.

64. Terry M. Shire kills Baxalta's hemophilia B program; clears path for BioMarin, Spark Therapeutics and uniQure. Available at: https://www.biospace.com/article/shire-kills-baxalta-s-hemophilia-b-program-clears-path-for-biomarin-spark-therapeutics-and-uniqure-/. Accessed August 4, 2016.

65. Semedo D. Dimension to end development of DTX101 as gene therapy for hemophilia B. Available at: https://hemophilianewstoday.com/2017/05/15/dimension-therapeutics-to-end-hemophilia-b-gene-therapy-dtx101-development/. Accessed May 15, 2017.

66. Gatlin A. Why analysts remain bullish on this hemophilia gene-therapy play. Available at: https://www.investors.com/news/technology/biomarin-pharmaceutical-hemophilia-a-gene-therapy/. Accessed May 22, 2018.

67. Pagliarulo N. Spark sheds $1B in value on hemophilia gene therapy data. Available at: https://www.biopharmadive.com/news/spark-gene-therapy-hemophilia-data-stock/529526/. Accessed August 7, 2018.

68. Herzog RW. A cure for hemophilia: the promise becomes a reality. Mol Ther 2016; 24:1503–4.

69. Sender R, Fuchs S, Milo R. Revised estimates for the number of human and bacteria cells in the body. PLoS Biol 2016;14:e1002533.

Moving?

Make sure your subscription moves with you!

To notify us of your new address, find your **Clinics Account Number** (located on your mailing label above your name), and contact customer service at:

Email: journalscustomerservice-usa@elsevier.com

800-654-2452 (subscribers in the U.S. & Canada)
314-447-8871 (subscribers outside of the U.S. & Canada)

Fax number: 314-447-8029

Elsevier Health Sciences Division
Subscription Customer Service
3251 Riverport Lane
Maryland Heights, MO 63043

*To ensure uninterrupted delivery of your subscription, please notify us at least 4 weeks in advance of move.

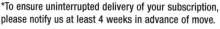